Autopsy of a Pandemic

The Lies, the Gamble, and the Covid-Zero Con

Julius Ruechel

To Dr. John Ioannidis,
whose bravery to stand firm against the tide of public opinion
helped me find my way back from the edge of fear and gives me
hope that science can be saved from what it has become.

And in memory of Nancy Russell,
who chose to end her life through assisted suicide
rather than endure the forced isolation of a second lockdown.
Lest we forget.

Table of Contents

Introduction: "Houston, We Have a Problem."

I heard the first rumblings of a new virus in China in late December of 2019. As those rumblings grew, I was initially quite alarmed. The anecdotes coming out of China were scary. Leaked video footage from China started circulating on social media, seemingly confirming the anecdotal stories. Then the numbers started trickling out. They were even more scary. And then all hell broke loose in Italy with devastating scenes of overflowing hospitals.

Yet throughout this early period, politicians and media in western countries seemed to systematically downplay the risk and ignore the medical professionals who were trying to raise the alarm — media and political attention were still wholly consumed by their effort to stoke a moral hysteria against President Trump. So, I began to dig into the data in order to try to gauge the threat coming towards us. And the numbers kept getting scarier.

In late January of 2020 many Chinese Canadians traveled to China to celebrate the Chinese New Year, including to Hubei province and to the city of Wuhan at the epicenter of the outbreak. As they returned, other Chinese-Canadians who had not traveled to China began to raise the alarm because they understood the significance of Chinese New Year (it is the largest annual migration of people in the world with close to 3 billion trips logged in China as people travel across the country to celebrate with their families), how it is celebrated (with huge festivals), and the vast scale of travelers that would be flying back and forth between China and Canada to participate in those celebrations. They recognized that an emerging epidemic happening during this critical season was creating the perfect storm to rapidly spread the virus all around the world. Many of these Chinese Canadians began to publicly speak out to ask those returning from the epicenter of the epidemic to self-isolate for a few days upon coming home in order to avoid spreading the virus in their communities and schools.

Canadian politicians and the media pounced on those raising the alarm but conveniently left out the ethnicity of those raising concerns and stripped their concerns of all context. Instead, they denounced these concerns as naked racism against Asian people, which meshed well with the go-to rhetoric used by politicians and media in their crusade against President Trump and his supporters. Race-baiting has long been a favorite political tool used by politicians to stoke division in order to portray themselves as the antidote — our Canadian Prime Minister, Justin Trudeau, has turned this strategy into an artform during his reign.

The Chinese Communist Party (CCP) also jumped on board the emerging narrative of racism in its eagerness to insulate itself from criticism over its role in the emerging outbreak. A totalitarian regime's greatest fear is crowds rising up against the government in anger. The CCP's handling of the virus left a lot to be angry about. Suppression of facts. Slow response. The giant Chinese New Year Party that party officials held in the city of Wuhan. Allowing over 5 million residents from Wuhan to scatter outside of the city at the beginning of the outbreak, thereby carrying the virus with them to all parts of China and to the rest of the world. And then there were the optics of the government-run Wuhan Institute of Virology, a level 4 biosafety laboratory conducting gain-of-function research on coronaviruses, which just happened to be located at the epicenter of the outbreak.

President Trump's decision to halt all travel from China on January 31st, 2020, only added fuel to the fire. At that point it became clear that the media and many politicians around the world were not just incompetent and ignoring the threat of the virus but were actively seeking to weaponize the outbreak as a political tool to paint President Trump and his supporters as xenophobic. And the CCP was learning to exploit the situation with wave after wave of well-timed face-saving propaganda to try to paint itself as the hero and not as the villain in the eyes of its own people and in the eyes of the world.

My wife and I prepared ourselves for the virus to arrive, tried warning family and friends of the growing threat, and stocked up on toilet paper. We were ready to weather a storm. Meanwhile, the majority of the world (outside of the medical community and a small minority of channels on social media) still seemed utterly oblivious to the threat that we were watching roll towards us in real time. We hunkered down to wait it out and tried (unsuccessfully) to convince our loved ones to do the same. They thought we were nuts because media and politicians were largely ignoring it and spinning concerns as evidence of racism.

Visions of the 1918 Spanish Flu and the medieval Plague filled our heads. Everyone else wanted to talk about President Trump. The numbers kept getting scarier. John Hopkins University put up its infamous COVID death-count dashboard that would eventually ensnare every eyeball in the world. Outbreaks began happening on cruise ships, like on the *Diamond Princess* cruise ship. Stories and images from Italy got worse. Slowly the world began to take notice.

But feeling prepared for the oncoming storm gave us room to think and the space to start to gain perspective. As the fear gradually spread through the rest of society, we watched many formerly independent thinkers, scientists, and academics (people that I once respected) as they began to launch vicious character-smearing attacks against the few lone voices in the medical community who were emerging with evidence-based challenges to the narrative of a dangerous global pandemic. I also initially thought the challengers were missing the obvious – couldn't they see the terrifying numbers on the COVID dashboard being published by John Hopkins University? Couldn't they see what was happening on cruise ships and in Italian hospitals?

A pivotal example was that of Dr. John Ioannidis, a world-leading biostatistician from Stanford University. I saw the flood of condemnation launched against Dr. Ioannidis in March of 2020 when he published his shockingly low infection fatality rate estimate, which essentially placed COVID in line with a bad winter flu (STAT News, March 17, 2020). I had never heard of Dr. Ioannidis. I looked at the John Hopkins COVID dashboard, convinced myself there must be something wrong with Dr. Ioannidis' thinking, and moved on. But the attacks launched against Dr. Ioannidis only grew louder, more vicious, and more personal. And I noticed that no-one was engaging with his data or providing meaningful counterevidence. It all amounted to little more than name-calling and character assassination. And it was being done by people with scientific backgrounds who should know better. That is not how science works.

If Dr. Ioannidis was going to flush his career down the drain by saying something blatantly stupid, I found it honorable that he was at least willing to provide the evidence to back up his claims. And I found it bizarre that his scientific peers were behaving like a pathetic university cancel culture mob instead of simply posting the data to disprove his claims. Cherry-picking studies that support preferred beliefs without wrestling with the data or the questions raised by conflicting studies is not how science works.

There is no idea so bad that it does not deserve to be demolished with evidence. There is no idea so righteous that it should be shielded from good-faith debate. Evidence and debate, not slander and deplatforming, are the currencies that make science work.

Dr. Ioannidis was willing to do his part. His critics were not. It made me mad. Considering the tsunami of public condemnation bearing down on him, I was struck by Dr. Ioannidis' unwavering courage to stand strong. It made me decide to take a closer look at his claims.

I hunted down the *Diamond Princess* cruise ship data (for example: WattsUpWithThat.com, March 16, 2020, and JudithCurry.com, March 25, 2020) as well as the follow-up paper Dr. Ioannidis' co-authored in April (Bendavid et al., 2020) and dug into the evidence. There was a lot of it. And it made sense. It raised questions in my mind. It made me recognize that there were a lot of people on a crusade to silence anyone raising evidence-based questions. It made me recognize the degree to which key medical concepts were being purposefully misrepresented by high level public health officials in their public discussion of the pandemic. It made me lose a lot of respect for a lot of people. And it made me realize that something was very very wrong within the medical community. It's what prompted me to start tracking down raw data instead of trusting the pre-digested pulp put out by official channels, which was being stripped of context for maximum fear-inducing effect.

Trust no-one. Verify everything. Science is not a battle of credentials, nor a belief in experts. Credentials are for job applications; they are irrelevant to the quest for knowledge. Science is a full contact sport that depends on evidence-based debate and everyone, no matter how humble, gets to participate as long as they do not try to exempt themselves from the burden of proof or shield themselves from their critics.

That was also the time period when I recognized the contemptable game being played with medical definitions, such as the confusion being created by mixing up population mortality, infection fatality rates, and case fatality rates. Comparisons were made with the Spanish Flu. It had a mortality rate of around 2.5%. By contrast, based on the initial Chinese and Italian data, the World Health Organization announced that COVID had a case fatality rate of 3.4%! A bigger number must be bad, right? But it's like comparing apples to oranges. A mortality rate of 2.5% meant that 2.5% of the entire world's population died. But digging into the history of the

Spanish Flu shows that only about a third of the world's population in 1918 became infected (500 million people), of which approximately 50 million died. So, in reality, the *infection* fatality rate of the Spanish Flu was much higher at around 10%.

And how does a 10% infection fatality rate compare with the WHO's initial COVID case fatality rate of 3.4%? A case and an infection are two very different things. Every case counts as an infection. Not every infection counts as a case.

In a pre-COVID world, a "case" used to describe an infected person who comes down with symptomatic disease (a.k.a. a sick person). An asymptomatic infection (a.k.a. a healthy person) didn't count as a case unless their infection actually led them to get sick. Only people with symptoms of sickness were counted as "cases". And only symptomatic people used to get PCR tests. By contrast, although sick people are counted as "infections", an infection also includes any asymptomatic person whose immune system fends off the virus without getting sick. Asymptomatic people would never previously have qualified for mass population-wide PCR testing. Broadly speaking, when a case fatality rate is calculated correctly, it essentially tells you what percentage of sick (symptomatic) people being admitted to hospital with disease will end up dying. By contrast, an infection fatality rate tells you what percentage of all people exposed to the virus (including those whose infections are mild or asymptomatic) will end up dying. Apples and oranges.

That's why (when you use the vocabulary correctly) you can have a virus that produces a very high case fatality rate but also has a very low infection fatality rate. Consider, for example, the case of the herpes virus. The WHO estimates that 67% of the global population under the age of 50 (3.7 billion people) are infected with herpes simplex virus type 1 (HSV-1) and a further 417 million people worldwide (11%) are infected by herpes simplex virus type 2 (HSV-2). In other words, herpes infections are everywhere. Now let me give you some case fatality rates for herpes: The case fatality rate of neonatal herpes (caused by either HSV-1 or HSV-2) is 60%. And the case fatality rate of herpes viral encephalitis (when one of these two herpes viruses reaches the brain) is 30% with treatment and 70-80% without treatment. Those are really scary numbers! Based on these case fatality rates, the herpes virus is extremely lethal, right? Nope. The WHO estimates that globally there are only 14,000 deaths per year of neonatal herpes and only approximately 15,000 cases of herpes viral encephalitis each year. In other words, while herpes is very dangerous for those who develop symptoms of neonatal herpes or herpes viral encephalitis, most people who are infected by herpes are not developing symptoms of either of these two dangerous diseases. The vast majority of people infected by HSV-1 get cold sores. And the vast majority of people infected by HSV-2 get genital herpes. Annoying, but certainly not deadly. With these numbers, it's safe to say that the overall infection fatality rate of the herpes virus is so small that it is statistically equivalent to zero despite the high case fatality rate among newborns or among people in which the virus reaches the brain.

Now consider what is being done during COVID. The headline "case fatality rate" of 3.4% that was initially promoted by the WHO was calculated using widespread PCR testing, which included testing many (but obviously not all) people with mild or no symptoms. So, the WHO's number was an utterly meaningless and dishonest number – a hybrid between a true case fatality rate and an infection fatality rate. It was data manipulation, custom-tailored to tell a lie. Public health agencies and the media all around the world have all repeated this sleight of hand despite knowing full well that it was an utterly dishonest and meaningless statistic.

Test more asymptomatic people and the hybrid number goes down. Test less asymptomatic people and the hybrid number goes up. By including some asymptomatic people in their PCR-testing, it inflated case numbers to give the impression that symptomatic disease was far more wide-spread that it actually was. But by stopping short of using antibody tests to calculate a proper infection fatality rate (as Dr. Ioannidis had done), they created the impression that the virus was far more deadly than it actually was. Dr. Ioannidis' early estimates were in the right ballpark and have stood the test of time. He and his colleagues have since used antibody testing to calculate an infection fatality rate of around 0.15% (Ioannidis, 2021). 0.15% is in the range of a bad winter flu season.

In other words, the Spanish Flu was almost 100 times more deadly than COVID. And during the Spanish Flu, the Grim Reaper preyed heavily on the young. During COVID, the Grim Reaper spends almost all his time stalking the corridors of nursing homes and palliative care homes where those with very weak immune systems live. Most children infected by the virus that causes COVID won't even know they've been infected unless someone shoves a Q-tip up their nose to collect the goop needed for a PCR test. Only those with severe pre-existing health conditions face any meaningful level of risk. Just like any other winter flu season.

In public discussions we use SARS-CoV-2 and COVID interchangeably, but it's actually wrong. SARS-CoV-2 is the name of the virus. COVID is the name of the disease caused by the virus *if someone gets sick*. An infection with the SARS-CoV-2 virus can either be asymptomatic (no disease) or lead to symptoms (COVID disease). A positive PCR test (or a positive antibody test) can only tell you whether you have a current or recent infection with the SARS-CoV-2 virus, but an infection does not necessarily mean you had COVID disease. Many people who are infected by the virus (and develop antibodies) never come down with the disease.

Referring to both the virus and the disease with the blanket term of "COVID" makes it easier to have a conversation about the pandemic — we all do it to make conversations flow better and I will continue to do so in this book for ease of reading — but by failing to make the distinction clear to the public, our public health officials, media, and politicians are obscuring the fact that the vast majority of infections do not lead to disease. The virus is far more widespread than you have been led to believe. But far less people came down with COVID disease than you have been led to believe.

Misrepresenting this fact created a tsunami of unnecessary panic. It's inexcusable.

As I recognized that those in charge were deliberately abusing vocabulary to stoke fear among unsuspecting citizens, it became clear that a repeat of the 2009 H1N1 Swine Flu debacle (or something like it) was unfolding. I will address this debacle in more detail later in the book but, broadly speaking, in 2009 our international public health organizations (led by the WHO), along with vaccine makers, used fear mongering, wildly inflated worst-case-scenario modelling, and shameless public manipulation to push a universal influenza vaccine on an unsuspecting public. Vaccine makers walked away with an additional $18 billion in revenues. As for the threat… despite all the hysteria, in the end the risk of serious illness was no higher than that of a regular seasonal flu.

Italy's lockdowns were another wake-up call for me. They demonstrated that the panic unleashed by the virus was motivating leaders in democratic countries to turn their backs on the long-standing fundamental principles of liberal democracy and embrace medieval impulses that strip individuals of their autonomy and of their human rights. Inalienable *individual* rights were invented as the antidote to government overreach – they are especially important during a crisis as checks and balances to set limits on what overzealous central planners can do to their citizens. Watching Italy suspend citizens' rights made me far more nervous than even the virus itself. Any society willing to suspend the individual human rights of its citizens to achieve "a greater good for the greatest number" is on its way to committing unspeakable monstrosities against some of its citizens.

In early March of 2020, still only partially awake to the unfolding scam, I warned a close family member not to take her family on a holiday outside of her local area for Spring Break just in case the virus washing up on our shores turned out to be deadly after all. And, even more importantly, I was deeply concerned that she might inadvertently getting caught on the wrong side of an Italian-style regional lockdown, which might prevent her from returning home if our politicians were to suddenly panic and bring lockdown hysteria to Canada. She shrugged it off and went on holiday anyways – our public health officials were still on TV telling everyone not to worry and not to cancel their Spring Break plans.

A week later (mid-March), I called this same family member after she returned home to let her know she was right not to worry, that the hysteria growing in the media was overblown, and to share the reality hidden in plain sight for anyone willing to dig through the government's own official data. My dive into the data had dissolved the last of my worries – the spell was broken. At that point I was still willing to give the government the benefit of the doubt that the hysteria was being driven by incompetence and not by malicious intent, but my alarm was gone.

But by then Sophie-Gregoire Trudeau (our Prime Minister's wife) had been publicly diagnosed with COVID, triggering a media frenzy that swept around the world. And the holiday town where my family member had stayed with her children during Spring Break had asked all holidaymakers to leave town, pronto. The appetite for medieval walls had arrived in Canada. And now our roles had reversed. Now she was caught up in the fear and playing catch up as the spell caught her in its web.

I had been worried when few around me were. Because I was early to the party, I had been trying to push a snowball uphill, facing a wall of indifference all the way. Because she was late to the party, she caught her fear just as everyone else was getting swept up in the same fear. Fear is contagious. Now the snowball was tumbling downhill with everyone working in unison to make it roll faster and grow larger. This was the seed for a bona fide self-reinforcing mass hysteria. Once again, I found myself pushing against the crowd, only now I faced outright hostility to my revised message.

Politicians and the media went so long denying the problem in its early days that when the public finally did take it seriously, it created a sudden switch from zero to maximum alarm. It caught everyone who had ignored the slow build up in January and February off guard. The sudden ramping up of alarm by the media, the media's fantastical predictions (like predictions that we might need ice hockey arenas to store the avalanche of corpses (National Post, March 14, 2020)), and contradictory public messaging from public health officials ("you don't need to wear a mask, we need them for health care workers") all served to amplify the hysteria, made the public feel like they'd been deceived, and left them scrambling in a mad dash for safety.

The media latched on to its new click-bait with great enthusiasm – this was far more potent even than stoking hysteria against President Trump as a tool to keep eyeballs glued to screens. And politicians suddenly found themselves on the defensive as their credibility was put in question after having ignored the problem for so long. They raced to get back out in front of the stampeding herd. Now no message of alarm was too extreme as long as it didn't provoke the anger of the crowd. Political survival is all about catering to the appetites of the crowd. Catering to a fearful crowd is like political manna from heaven.

And therein lies the trap. Fear is a blinding emotion. Once the media and politicians started beating the drums of hysteria, there was no way for anyone newly aware of the problem to gain perspective. The public became trapped in a desperate cycle of fear and fixated on the media and on public health officials as their path to safety.

People rushed to stock up their pantries and bolt their doors. Toilet paper shortages emerged, which only heightened the fear that we might be standing on the edge of a complete breakdown of civil society. Celebrities flocked to the cause, never shy to dramatize an issue. Naomi Campbell showed up at the airport wearing a hazmat suit, goggles, face mask, fashionable pink latex gloves, and carrying an arsenal of anti-bacterial wipes to disinfect everything in her path (CNN, March 11, 2020). Visions of the 1918 Spanish Flu and the medieval Plague consumed the public imagination. Meanwhile, the deeper I dove into the data, the clearer it was becoming that Dr.

Ioannidis was dead right. This virus was a giant nothingburger, a bad flu driven by a new strain of a well-known family of coronaviruses, dangerous to those with weak immune systems but otherwise a non-event for almost everyone else.

Once you gain perspective, it's easy to see through the fear and to catch the lies and manipulation. It's easy to see the players who deliberately stoke panic while making personal life choices which expose that they don't believe the narrative they are promoting. And it's easy to start digging to let the data tell its own story without getting caught up in the flood of blinding emotions that are being peddled on the 6 o'clock news.

I was fortunate that I had long since cancelled my cable TV subscription and was already in the habit of digging into the raw data on news stories without relying on the mainstream media to pre-digest that data for me. I was fortunate that I was exposed to the story so early that I was able to watch the slow build up in January and February without being surrounded by a bubble of contagious group fear. And I was fortunate that we had several months to prepare ourselves in case things turned into Italian-style lockdowns without having to compete with anyone else as we stockpiled food and toilet paper. It kept us from completely losing ourselves to blind panic. Instead, worry gradually dissolved into doubt, doubt gradually turned into perspective, and perspective motivated more deep dives into the data.

But for someone caught up in that abrupt unexpected mood shift in early March, suddenly confronted by an avalanche of media hysteria, suddenly confronted by public health officials putting on shameless drama presentations night after night, and suddenly finding themselves competing with other shoppers for toilet paper, it had a crippling effect. They were completely caught off balance. And the rapidly evolving situation, relentless lies, ever-changing rules, and the hysteria pushed by the very same people to whom citizens would inevitably turn for information on how to keep safe (the government and the media) created a near-impossible trap for anyone to easily climb out of. Unless someone either had first-hand knowledge of the lies, had long-standing knowledge about virology, or was personally harmed by the measures being rolled out by the government, they had little choice but to put their trust in the media, the leaders, and the "experts".

The natural place to turn during a time of crisis is to our leaders and to our scientific community for guidance on how to keep safe and, of course, to our media to provide impartial information. But when those pillars of democracy are compromised by partisan and opportunistic conflicts of interest, or by an agenda, it is a perfect recipe for a runaway self-feeding hysteria. It's hardly surprising that unfamiliar voices, like myself and the thousands (now millions) of others around the world, were ignored when we tried to pull the brakes. For people caught up in this trap, letting go of their trust in their leaders, public health officials, and mainstream media outlets would have made their fear even more intolerable. Having no-one to trust (or trusting completely unknown strangers) during a crisis is even more paralyzing than trusting flawed but familiar individuals and familiar institutions in positions of power. Seeking safety by aligning oneself with those who hold power over our lives is the psychological basis of how Stockholm Syndrome can turn captives into willing participants in their own hostage-taking.

As I saw the pillars of science and democracy give way to panic, medieval superstition, and authoritarian control, I was unable to stay silent on the sidelines. Mainstream media had clearly abandoned their responsibility to do objective investigative journalism, which is required to create transparency and put checks and balances on government overreach and institutional misconduct. There were so few voices pushing back to try to hold our leaders' feet to the fire.

I published my first article about COVID on my website on April 20th, 2020. It took me more than a month to amalgamate a coherent body of work based on the data being released by official government agencies and research being published in medical journals around the world. And I kept on writing as I tried to gain perspective on why our society was being swept down the rabbit hole into runaway mass hysteria despite all the clear medical evidence against it and despite all the constitutional protections and fundamental human rights that were meant to prevent this sort of descent into tyranny.

What follows in this book are my three most important data deep dives. For anyone caught up in the panic, they clear a path through the fog of chaos to help them break free from fear. For anyone who has broken free of the spell, they provide a kind of record to gain perspective over what has been done to us. And for future generations, I hope this book serves as a warning to prevent this from ever happening again.

Part one, *The Lies Exposed by the Numbers,* tells the story of the pandemic using the government's own official data. What emerges is a shocking story of deliberate scientific misconduct and breach of trust, which reveals the horrifying - and deadly - consequences of stripping data of context and allowing government to evade transparency.

A scandal of this global scale would require an entire Encyclopedia in order to expose everything in meaningful detail – anything less would require such broad generalizations that it would cease to be useful as an exposé. So, I have chosen to focus most closely on Canada in this section of the book to provide a digestible snapshot of what happened over the last year and a half. However, although there are slight differences in the numbers from one country to the next, the broader trend and the lessons learned from this deep dive apply equally to all countries. Some version of what happened in Canada, happened everywhere. Once you see it, you will recognize the same patterns and the same strategies in your own country.

Part two, *Washington's Inoculation Gamble,* focuses on the government's decision to rely on vaccines as an exit strategy. It demonstrates why the principle of informed consent has been systematically ignored. And it does what governments have refused to do: it uses the government's own numbers to calculate the Vegas odds of death from the virus versus the odds of injury or death from the vaccine – this simple calculation, along with the freedom to refuse any medical treatment, is essential to the principle of informed consent, which was established by the Nuremberg Code in the aftermath of the Second World War. Part two is designed to help you take back control over your medical decisions and give you the knowledge base to stop being manipulated by public health officials that are willfully distorting basic medical principles and using coercion to push universal vaccines as an exit strategy.

And in part three, *The Snake-Oil Salesmen and the Covid-Zero Con,* I take you on a tour though pre-COVID science to demonstrate that, from day one, the initial push for lockdowns and vaccines as an exit strategy were a deliberate fantasy that was cultivated by international health agencies and vaccine developers. It was a fantasy designed to rope us into a pharmaceutical dependency as a deceitful trade-off for access to our lives. Variant by variant. For as long as the public is willing to go along for the ride. It's the subscription-based business model, adapted to the pharmaceutical industry. "Immunity as a service". Combined with PCR testing, which costs between US$36 and US$180 a pop (with more than 615 million tests performed in the US alone by September 17th, 2021), this may be the world's most lucrative shakedown ever perpetrated on an unsuspecting public.

There are many additional layers to this pandemic: the psychological roots of the growing hysteria, the never-ending stream of opportunists capitalizing on the pandemic for their own benefit, the irreversible social-engineering initiatives that are being grafted onto society under the guise of public health, the creation of a two-tier society in the name of "public safety", the rapidly escalating demonization of convenient scapegoats, and the tyrannical police state that is emerging from the chaos. Those are the subjects of other essays, which you will find on my website at **www.juliusruechel.com**. But the first step towards dismantling the hysteria, regaining our freedom, reforming our scientific institutions, and reclaiming our liberal democracy is to be able to step back and see the pandemic from a birds-eye view. Once we all understand what was done to us and how we were manipulated into this position, we gain the ability to fight back.

Knowledge is power. It makes us immune to the cycle of fear. The magic trick loses its magic when the crowd understands the sleight of hand. Perspective gives us the strength to focus on the battles yet to come, which have little to do with the virus and everything to do with freeing ourselves from the medical tyranny and the cycle of fear that has consumed our nations.

When I write, I write to organize my thoughts. I hope reading these essays will help you regain your peace of mind as much as writing them have helped me maintain my sanity over these long dark months.

PART I —
The Lies Exposed by the Numbers: Fear, Misdirection, and Institutional Deaths

On April 30th, 2021, Canada published a weekly COVID-19 epidemiology report that included a simple breakdown of cases and deaths linked to outbreaks, organized according to the **location of the source of infection**. Beneath the unassuming superficial appearance of this data set lies the incriminating key to exposing (and prosecuting) a jaw dropping series of scandals.

Once the data is put into context, clear proof emerges that gross negligence on the part of government policymakers directly led to the preventable deaths of thousands, most especially among the most vulnerable that the government claims to be trying to protect. The data also makes it crystal clear why "two weeks to flatten the curve" turned into a never-ending year-and-a-half-long nightmare and why lockdowns as a public health strategy were a misbegotten fantasy that was doomed from the start.

The remarkable story told by the data exposes in almost comical relief just how shamefully the government whipped the public into fear by cultivating a sense of vulnerability that is entirely out of touch with reality. But the data set goes even further than that. Written in black and white in the government's own official numbers, published by the Public Health Agency of Canada, lies the evidence that the blame for much of the dying lies squarely in policymakers' hands for decisions taken on its turf, behind institutional walls, and not with the individual actions and choices made by citizens out in the broader community.

No matter how familiar you think you are with the chaos that has unfolded over the past year and a half, I guarantee you there are surprises in this investigative report for everyone. And I believe it contains the conclusive evidence to hold our leaders legally accountable for the lethal consequences of abandoning long-established pandemic protocols, which were meticulously documented in the WHO's 2019 pandemic planning guide (WHO, 2019) and which were specifically designed to prevent the epidemic of fear and DIY ad-hoc rule-making that have been on display throughout this crisis.

So, over the coming paragraphs I am going to take you on a guided tour through the pandemic, simply by providing context to the numbers. The tour starts slowly with revelations that you would expect if you have been paying attention over the past year and a half. But as the layers of evidence begin to stack up, one on top of the other, and as the implications of each layer become clear, the fog of the last year and a half of chaos will begin to lift. What emerges is a shocking story of scientific misconduct and breach of trust, which reveals the horrifying - and deadly - consequences of stripping data of context and allowing government to evade transparency.

I have laid out this horrifying story to help us all gain perspective, to serve as a tool to rescue loved ones from the government's shameless fearmongering, and to provide lawyers with a fully referenced framework, with links to original data sources throughout the text and/or in chart captions, to help them build cases to hold these people accountable for what they have done.

1 — Dr. Bonnie Henry Lands a Whopper: Not Every Lie Requires False Data to Tell a False Story.

One of the most powerful tools in a magician's toolkit is the art of misdirection: using flashy cues that naturally attract the public's eye in order to distract from that which the magician does not want you to see. But the most skilled masters of this art are politicians and public officials who use it to manipulate public opinion and distract from their own misdeeds. "Cases, cases, cases", anti-lockdown protests, anti-maskers, the pastors that opened their churches, the restaurant that refused to close - these convenient scapegoats are the noisy tools of misdirection exploited by our government throughout this crisis. Now I'm going to turn the camera angle to expose the illusion and show you what the magician has been trying so hard to prevent you from seeing.

I'm going to start this tour of the pandemic with a brief example of the kind of flagrant misrepresentation of data that has been utilized by health authorities and the media throughout this crisis. This example also introduces some of the key themes and background details that will accompany us throughout the rest of the scandal.

On April 19th, the Vancouver Sun published a story (Vancouver Sun, April 19th, 2021) about the COVID-linked death of an infant under two years old:

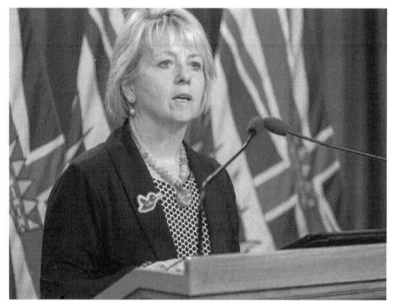

VANCOUVER SUN

Infant dies from COVID-19 at B.C. Children's Hospital

"It reminds us of the vicious nature of this virus," says provincial health officer Dr. Bonnie Henry

David Carrigg
Apr 19, 2021 • April 19, 2021 • 2 minute read • 💬 25 Comments

Premier John Horgan, Health Minister Adrian Dix and Chief Provincial Health Officer Dr. Bonnie Henry provide an update on COVID-19 on April 19, 2021. PHOTO BY SUBMITTED PHOTO, GOVERNMENT OF B /PNG

Figure 1: Dr. Henry referenced the death of an infant under 2 years old to remind everyone of *"the vicious nature of this virus."* Context was dangerously absent from this statement (Vancouver Sun, April 19th, 2021).

Dr. Bonnie Henry, BC's provincial health officer, took the opportunity to tell the public that the infant's tragic death "reminds us of the vicious nature of this virus." The fear sparked by the headline and by Dr. Bonnie Henry's statement is palpable. Yet buried in the text of the article is the missing context. Dr. Henry was using the magician's tool of misdirection to hide what was in plain sight.

Latest data from the B.C. Centre for Disease Control shows that as of April 3 there had been 52 hospital admissions for people aged under 10 in B.C., and four of those cases were in intensive care. The child's death is the first in anyone in B.C. under the age of 30.

Figure 2: Excerpt from the Vancouver Sun article in figure 1.

The very same article goes on to say that this was the very first death under the age of 30 in the entire province of British Columbia (population 5 million)! More than a year (and two waves) into the pandemic! That in itself highlights just how NOT dangerous this virus is to young people under the age 30.

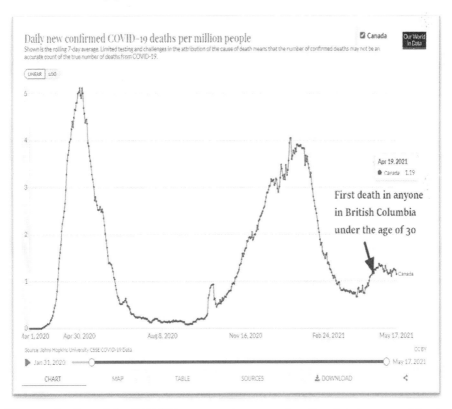

Figure 3: Canada's COVID waves (not much of a third wave either), showing the date of BC's first death of anyone under the age of 30. (Our World in Data, May 7th, 2021)

To illustrate this point further, let's compare COVID deaths in children (0-19) to influenza and pneumonia deaths in children (0-19). Over the first 15 months of the COVID pandemic, a total of 11 children (age 0 to 19 years) died of COVID in all of Canada (population 38 million). By contrast, as figure 4 demonstrates, an average of 25 children (age 0 to 19 years) die of influenza and pneumonia every year:

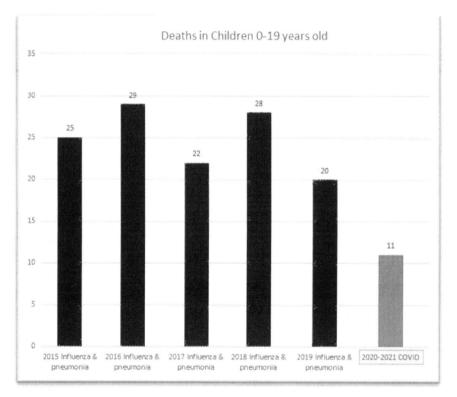

Figure 4: Comparing COVID deaths to influenza and pneumonia deaths in children aged 0 to 19 years of age. (Statistics Canada, May 20th, 2021) and Government of Canada daily epidemiology report for May 7th, 2021. (Government of Canada, May 8th, 2021)

Now consider a few other tidbits hidden in the meat of the article, which directly contradict the frightening impression given by the headline and by Dr. Henry's statement.

An infant under two years of age has died from COVID-19 at B.C. Children's Hospital, becoming the youngest person to die from the disease in Canada.

The provincial health officer said the infant lived in the Fraser Health region but was being treated at the hospital in Vancouver and had another health problem.

Figure 5: Excerpt from the Vancouver Sun article in figure 1.

This infant caught its infection inside the BC Children's Hospital. It was already a patient before catching the virus. It was a hospital-transmitted infection, not an infection caught at school or out in the community. It was an infection caught behind the doors of a government institution. This matters because it reveals that the infant was not an average healthy child living as part of the regular community but rather that it already had extremely serious pre-existing health conditions, which were so severe that it required seeking out specialized care.

"Although this child had pre-existing health conditions that complicated their illness, it was the virus that caused their death," Henry said. "It reminds us of the vicious nature of this virus."

Figure 6: Excerpt from the Vancouver Sun article in figure 1.

Kids do not go to the BC Children's Hospital because they break their arms or come down with chickenpox. The BC Children's Hospital uniquely specializes in treating only the most seriously ill or injured children from across British Columbia (Provincial Health Services Authority. n.d.). Their focus is on providing specialty services found nowhere else in the province. Yet this infant travelled outside of its own health region to receive "specialized care at the BC Children's Hospital in Vancouver" (CTV News, April 19th, 2021). Its pre-existing conditions must have been serious indeed if the services it required were not available in its own health region.

Yet the article neglects to mention what pre-existing conditions the infant had and Dr. Henry goes out of her way to emphasize that it was the virus and not the pre-existing conditions that led to its death. This deflects from being able to understand what role these pre-existing conditions played in increasing the infant's vulnerability to the COVID virus. And then she immediately misdirects attention elsewhere by following up with a generic statement about risk from the virus ("the vicious nature of the virus"), which makes everyone recoil in fear and imagine the risks to themselves and their own children.

It was a magician's masterful use of misdirection to distract from the actual important facts of this story while heightening everyone's sense of vulnerability. She succeeded in telling exactly the opposite story told by the facts. She hijacked this infant's tragic death to craft an entirely different public message. And her message is difficult to criticize without coming off like a heartless monster that minimizes this infant's tragic death.

Linking the sad fate of this infant to the risk posed to the other 1.7 million children and young adults under 30 (Statistics Canada, July 6th, 2021) living in the province is an unconscionable abuse of her authority and a dereliction of her duty to accurately educate the public of its risks. She spread misinformation by creating a false impression of what the underlying facts mean, by emphasizing and dramatizing some facts using extremely fear-inducing language, by withholding context, and by de-emphasizing the most important parts of the story. A lie created without actually falsifying any data.

It was a lie worthy of a Pinocchio Award. But it is tiny compared to the big scandal that this investigative report is really about. And, as you shall soon see as the details of this scandal become clear, if Dr. Henry is right that the virus and not the infant's pre-existing conditions were the ultimate cause of its death, then this infant's tragic death was most probably preventable had the government not turned its back on the WHO's pandemic planning guidelines (WHO, 2019) 15 months earlier.

Now I recommend that you go get yourself a cup of coffee and find someplace comfortable to sit. Because clearing a path through a year-and-a-half-long scandal takes more than a few paragraphs, but I promise it will be worth every minute of your time.

2 — A Little Housekeeping: Opening Statements

Before I begin untangling this scandalous web of lies, here is Health Canada's official definition of an outbreak, just so we are all on the same page as the conversation switches back and forth between deaths linked to outbreaks versus deaths that are not linked to outbreaks:

COVID-19 Outbreak: Two or more confirmed cases of COVID-19 epidemiologically linked to a specific setting and/or location. Excluding households, since household cases may not be declared or managed as an outbreak if the risk of transmission is contained. This definition also excludes cases that are geographically clustered (e.g. in a region, city, or town) but not epidemiologically linked, and cases attributed to community transmission.

Figure 7: Outbreak - official definition used by Health Canada (Government of Canada, 2021)

And here is a screenshot of the incriminating outbreak data set, which organizes all 13,789 outbreak-linked deaths by their source of infection. This is the data I am about to put into context, layer by layer. And rest assured, by the time I reach the end of this story all the other 10,613 deaths not linked to outbreaks will also fall into place. They too are an essential part of the larger scandal that I am about to expose.

COVID-19 IN CANADA

Table 6. Total number of COVID-19 outbreaks, cases, and deaths by outbreak setting in Canada as of 24 April 2021[a]

Outbreak setting	Total number of outbreaks reported	Total number of cases reported	Total number of reported deaths	Outbreaks reported during week 16
Community[b]	229	15 181	141	3
Corrections/shelter/congregate living	796	14 455	226	30
Food/drink/retail	756	3 013	3	11
Healthcare	850	11 134	844	19
Industrial (including agricultural)[c]	651	14 903	25	35
Long term care and retirement residences	4 643	67 806	12 541	56
Personal Care[d]	61	747	0	0
School & Childcare Centre[e]	1 548	9 016	1	33
Other[f]	664	6 017	8	21

Source: Publicly reported outbreak data, including Provincial and Territorial websites.
Note: These categories include both current and retrospective outbreak data.
[a] This is not an all-inclusive list and is subject to change based on current and active outbreak locations reported.
[b] Community includes population centres, Indigenous communities, Mennonite, Reserves, and small city outbreaks.
[c] The number of outbreaks in Windsor-Essex have been grouped into one cluster; industrial settings include: automotive manufacturing, distribution/processing facilities, worker camps, waste management/recycling, warehouse, etc.
[d] Personal care refers to personal care services, such as hair salons, nail salons, etc.
[e] Child and youth care include daycare centres and day camps; excludes any facilities that report only one case. Schools with only one case, or those for which information on number of cases is unknown, have been excluded.
[f] Other groups together outbreaks in settings not listed in the categories above, for example social gatherings, office workplaces, recreational facilities, etc.

Figure 8: The original data: outbreaks by setting. Canada COVID-19 Weekly epidemiology report, published April 30th, 2021 (Public Health Agency of Canada, April 30th, 2021)

3 — How Big are Outbreaks in Different Settings?

The first layer of this story, represented by figure 9 below, uses the outbreak data to show the average number of cases involved in each outbreak, based on the setting where each infection took place.

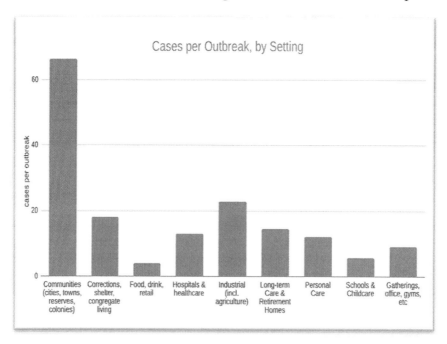

Figure 9: Average number of cases per outbreak (reported cases ÷ reported outbreaks). A tall column = large outbreaks. A short column = small outbreaks). From data shown in figure 8. Calculations in the Notes[1].

As you can see, the largest outbreaks are community spread. The average outbreak in enclosed settings like schools, restaurants, gyms and even long-term care facilities is smaller than outbreaks caused by just living life in general. It becomes clear that places like schools, restaurants, gyms, and retail stores do NOT cause larger outbreaks than any other settings despite being the focus of much of the government's ad-hoc rule making.

If anything, restaurants, schools, gyms, and retail stores produce the *smallest* cluster of cases if an outbreak does occur.

But there is one category that should really spark your curiosity because it is missing altogether. Travel.

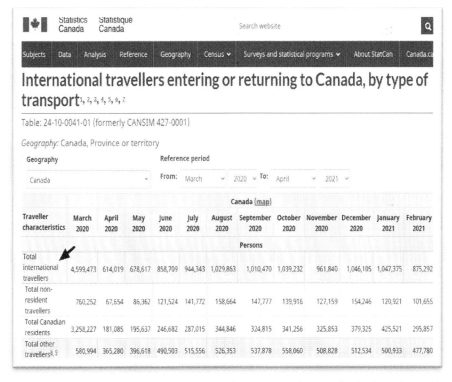

Figure 10: More than 4.5 million travelers entered Canada during the rush home in March of 2020. Another 10 million entered the country between April 2020 and February 2021. Yet travel did not cause sufficient outbreaks to warrant its own category in the outbreak data set. (Statistics Canada, July 6th, 2021)

Where are the travel-linked outbreaks? Despite more than 4.5 million travelers entering Canada during the peak rush to come home in March of 2020. Despite more than 10 million travelers, an average of over 900,000 per month (!), entering Canada in a steady stream ever since. Despite a significant portion our political classes having travelled to the Caribbean over the winter holidays while Canada remained trapped in lockdown. Despite the lack of social distancing on airplanes. Despite the millions of travelers who were crammed together at border checkpoints as they waited to get through airport customs and receive medical screenings at the start of the pandemic when the government asked millions of Canadians to all come home, all at once (remember the photos and the outrage in the news?). And despite all those travelers at the start of the pandemic not wearing masks or social distancing because at that time the government had not yet decided that they were a thing (more on that later).

Yet travel did not even warrant its own category as a source of outbreaks!

This is the first of a long list of clues exposing how health officials and media have encouraged fearful beliefs about the behavior of this virus, which are completely out of sync with the story told by the government's own numbers.

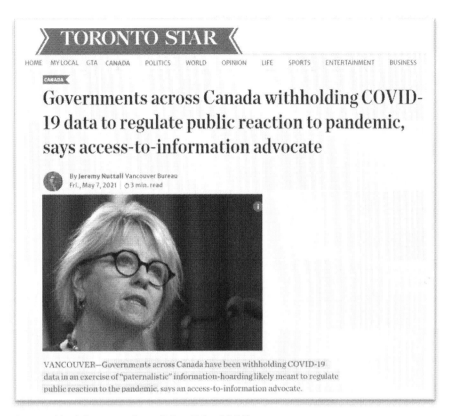

Figure 11: (Toronto Star, May 7th, 2020)

But while the location of infections is clearly not playing a big role in the *size* of outbreaks, there is a huge difference to how *deadly* outbreaks are in different settings. Not all outbreaks are created equal. The next chapter is where the story starts to get interesting and population-wide really lockdowns start to fall apart.

4 — How Deadly are Outbreaks in Different Settings?

This next chart looks at how deadly an outbreak is likely to be if it occurs in different settings. It shows the average number of deaths linked to each individual outbreak in each of these various locations.

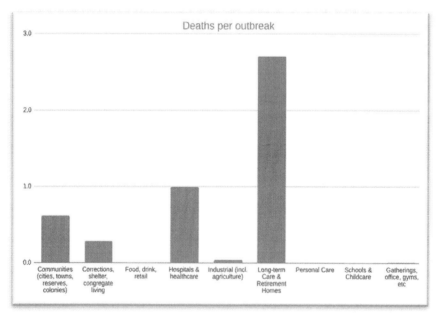

Figure 12: Deaths per outbreak (reported deaths ÷ reported outbreaks). Not every setting has the same kind of people in it. Tall columns are places where high-risk people hang out. Short columns are places where low-risk people hang out. From data shown in figure 8. Calculations in the Notes[1].

As you would expect, outbreaks in long-term care facilities and hospitals are much more dangerous (more deaths per outbreak) than outbreaks in the rest of community. Outbreaks in schools, gyms, restaurants, processing plants, personal care, and so on are essentially irrelevant to your statistical risk of dying because there are so few deaths linked to infections caught in these settings. A PCR-confirmed case does not automatically unleash the Hellhounds to snap at your heels. The level of risk in different settings are orders of magnitude apart.

Of course, that shouldn't surprise us. Residents in long-term care facilities and patients in hospitals are obviously *much* more vulnerable than the rest of the population because *they already have severe pre-existing diseases and/or severely weakened immune systems*. **They wouldn't be hanging out in these settings if they weren't already sick and vulnerable *before* catching COVID.**

I have highlighted this seemingly obvious statement because it is an important building block to understand the eye-popping layers that come later in this story. It foreshadows the first glimpse of the scandal, which will become clear and clearer as the layers add up.

5 — If You Get Infected, What Is Your Chance of Dying?

Another way to look at the outbreak data is to look at what percentage of infections (i.e. cases confirmed by a PCR test) will lead to death in each setting. It reinforces what was clearly shown in the previous chapter. Infections in different settings lead to very different outcomes.

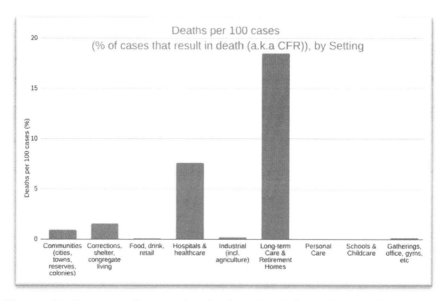

Figure 13: Percent of cases that lead to death in outbreaks, by setting. (reported deaths ÷ reported cases x 100). Tall columns = high risk of death. Short columns = low risk of death. From data shown in figure 8. Calculations in the Notes[1].

It takes very few infections to lead to an outbreak-linked death in a long-term care facility (1 in 5). But boatloads of people can be infected in nail salons (no outbreak deaths), restaurants (1 in 1004), churches, gyms, and stores (1 in 752), and schools (1 in 9016) while producing next to zero fatalities. Living your life is not dangerous. Having a severe pre-existing health condition or a severely compromised immune system are necessary pre-requisites before you have cause to worry.

Those who face a high risk of dying of COVID are those who are already so sick and/or so restricted in their ability to move about their community that very few of them are actually visiting any of these other locations. In other words, those who are extremely vulnerable are already so sickly or so incapacitated *before* catching COVID that the majority most of them do not go to gyms, restaurants, churches, or nail salons. If they did, these settings would not have so few outbreak-linked deaths. *Their pre-existing health conditions are so severe that their health conditions are effectively filtering them from the rest of the community and keeping them bottled up at home or in health care facilities.*

Assessing your personal level of risk from this virus begins by understanding the story told by the simple chart in figure 13. It highlights that people with pre-existing conditions face a *much* higher risk of death if they are infected by the SARS-CoV-2 virus than everyone else. The sheer size difference between columns should start making anyone not familiar with these numbers start to sit up and take notice. Let's quantify those differences.

6 — Relative Risk: Not All Outbreaks Are Created Equal

The different heights of the columns in the previous graph illustrate the difference of risk in different settings. The eye-popping realizations begin when we start crunching the numbers to see just how big the difference actually is. *It's absolutely mindbogglingly enormous!* Yet this nuanced detail is almost universally absent from the public messaging surrounding this virus.

- For example: an infection at a school is **1,668** times LESS likely to result in death than an infection at a long-term care facility and **683** times LESS likely to result in death than an infection at a hospital. This virus is not a vicious beast preying on children. It is the Grim Reaper calling early on those already teetering on death's door.

- A less awkward way of expressing this it is that restaurants are 186 times safer than long-term care facilities and 76 times safer than hospitals.

- Gyms are 139 times safer than a long-term care facility and 57 times safer than hospitals.

- Working in a meat processing facility is 110 times safer than being a resident at a long-term care facility and 45 times safer than being a patient at a hospital.

Common sense tells us that it is not the buildings themselves that change the level of personal risk in each of these settings but rather that it is the specific characteristics of the people who are hanging out in them. To a large extent, that's true, but only up to a point. As you will soon see once we get to the meat of this scandal, some of the buildings involved in these outbreaks (and specifically the terrible decisions being made by those who manage these buildings) are actually the most significant part of this whole scandal. Vulnerability + bad management = death. As you will see as the story continues to unfold, infections that result in death almost always require both of these ingredients. One is rarely enough.

For those who would like to play with the math themselves to compare risks in different settings, here are the raw numbers from the previous graph: One-size-fits-all policymaking is ridiculous when different demographics have such different levels of risk.

Setting	Deaths per 100 cases (%)
Communities (cities, towns, reserves, colonies)	0.928793
Corrections, shelter, congregate living	1.563473
Food, drink, retail	0.099569
Hospitals & healthcare	7.580384
Industrial (incl. agriculture)	0.167751
Long-term Care & Retirement Homes	18.495413
Personal Care	0.000000
Schools & Childcare	0.011091
Gatherings, office, gyms, etc	0.132957

Figure 14: Deaths per 100 cases (a.k.a. Case Fatality Rate), by setting. From data shown in figure 8, calculations in the Notes[1].

This was the tip of the iceberg...

7 — Why Are So Few People Dying Outside of Institutions?

I think we can agree by now that when the virus goes on the hunt, it is finding different kinds of prey in different settings. The most vulnerable prey are those living in long-term care homes as well as patients in hospitals who already suffer from other serious pre-existing conditions, like Alzheimer's, dementia, cancer, or leukemia.

Children, office workers, mall shoppers, personal care clients, gym-goers, restaurant guests, and industrial workers rarely have such severe life-threatening pre-existing conditions that they become easy prey for this virus. The virus can infect them. But the overwhelming majority of these encounters have a happy ending. A *significant* number of them will not even experience a single disease symptom (Washington Post, August 8th, 2020). Mild pre-existing conditions, which many active people in the community have, are not a death sentence. Severity matters.

So how many of the total outbreak-linked deaths are from infections caught in these two high-risk settings: long-term care and hospitals?

Hold on to your hat... a full *97% of outbreak-related deaths are in* **long-term care and hospitals/healthcare**!

Add **prison** populations and that number rises to a full **98.6%**!

And I promise, you'll soon understand why I have chosen to add prisons to this select group of settings.

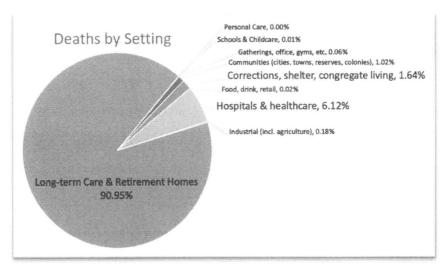

Figure 15: Outbreak-linked deaths by setting: 98.6% of deaths are linked to outbreaks in just three settings: long-term care facilities, hospitals, and prisons. From data shown in figure 8. Calculations in the Notes[1].

The remarkable pie chart in figure 15 begins to put the risk to the general public into perspective. Anyone not hanging out in one of these three settings faces an almost inconsequentially small level of risk from this virus.

The pie chart demonstrates that this is a crisis that affects people with extremely serious pre-existing health conditions and compromised immune systems. *And almost no-one else.*

But if you think you're beginning to gain perspective, I haven't even started getting to the good bits yet. Remember, there are also large numbers of people with equally serious pre-existing health conditions and compromised immune systems living *outside* of these three settings, but they are *not* dying in droves.

Why are the vulnerable living *outside* of these three institutions not suffering the same fate? The eye-popping layers of this scandal begin here...

8 — Captive Populations vs The Rest of the Community

If you thought that 98.6% number was surprising (it surprised the heck out of me, which is why I started digging deeper into this particular outbreak data set in the first place), I'd now like to point out exactly what these three settings are. The people in these unique settings are essentially *captive* populations that are *permanently or semi-permanently segregated from the rest of society* **inside government-owned or government-regulated institutions**. (Note: Privately-run nursing homes fall under this category because they are extremely tightly regulated by the government in order to acquire and maintain their licenses. They are privately owned, but they operate according to the government's rules.)

All three are *institutional* settings. Everyone who lives in these three settings is either a resident, a patient, or a prisoner. They don't go home at night. They don't mix with the rest of the population. They live there, permanently or semi-permanently. The only way they get to mingle with us is if *we* visit them. And we are only allowed in after staff members look us over, test us, and let us through the door. The people inside these settings already *live behind an institutional wall*. They permanently live under some form of lockdown, even when the rest of society does not.

I'm going to say it one more time, because it's so important to everything else that comes next:

They already live behind an institutional wall — they are permanently in some form of lockdown, even when we are not.

48

Which means that, despite all the shaming about our desire to have a BBQ in our backyards with our friends, 98.6% of outbreak-linked deaths are from infections caught and spread *inside* the walls of tightly controlled institutional environments, not out in the community.

For the past year and a half these institutions have been closed or severely restricted to the public. If the virus makes it in, it is because staff brought the virus with them to work or when health officials transferred patients from hospitals *into* long-term care in order to free up hospital beds (Globe and Mail, April 22nd, 2021). !?!

There is an equivalent of a medieval wall separating the people living inside these institutions from those living outside these walls. Their world and our world are permanently separated by an institutional barrier. There is a door that leads between these two worlds, *but the government has the option to close that door, even to seal it, at any time.*

As long as the government defends that institutional barrier between our two parallel worlds whenever there is a virus circulating outside, the rules imposed on those living outside are largely irrelevant to those living inside. These institutions were designed to function that way. During bad winter flu seasons, staff of long-term care homes have the option to shut the doors and live on the inside with their patients (McKnight's Long-term Care News, August 18th, 2020) for a few weeks while the worst of the flu surge passes through the population outside.

Pandemics, like winter flu season, tend to come in waves, each of which tend to last around 6 to 8 weeks, give or take, and then the doors can be reopened. The waves shown earlier in figure 3 are a good example.

That is how long it takes for most respiratory viruses to surge through a healthy population when general population-wide lockdowns are not used to slow the spread. But "flattening the curve" stretches that 6-to-8-week period into months, now over a year and a half, and there still isn't enough natural immunity built up outside the walls to safely reopen the doors between these two separate worlds. Isolation kills in its own right. And defending a door for 18 uninterrupted months all but guarantees a steady stream of mishaps that let the virus through the door (more on that later).

98.6% of *all* outbreak-linked deaths are the result of infections caught *inside* these institutional barriers. Only 1.4% are linked to outbreaks in the community at large. That context is probably starting to grow a queasy feeling in the pit of your stomach about how this pandemic is being managed. But this is just the beginning of the scandal.

9 — Institutionalized People, the Community on the Outside, and the Wall That Divides them

I'm going to reorganize the data from the pie chart in figure 15. I'm regrouping all those deaths into two very simple categories because this important distinction sets the stage for the next set of big eye-popping revelations:

- **Institutionalized People** (deaths in tall column)
- **The Rest of Us (Community)** (deaths in short column)

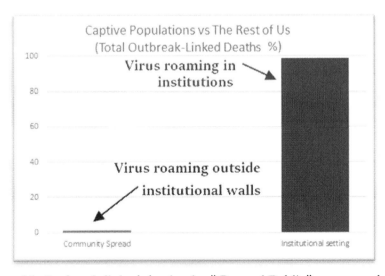

Figure 16: Outbreak-linked deaths the "General Public" versus outbreak-linked deaths among people living in institutionalized settings (i.e. long-

term care, hospitals, prisons). From data shown in figure 8. Calculations in the Notes[1].

At this point of the story, I'm sure it has become quite clear just how specific this crisis is. Despite the fact that the virus is clearly circulating on both sides of that institutional barrier, the vast majority of the deaths are linked to infections spreading on only one side of that barrier. This is not a general population crisis; it is an institutional crisis.

Figure 17 provides another perspective on what is happening on either side of that institutional divide.

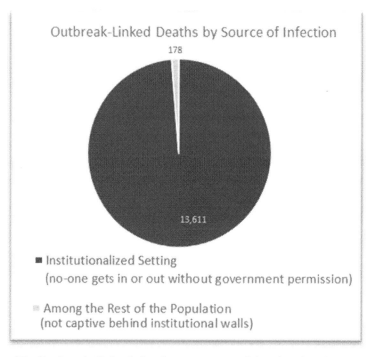

Figure 17: Outbreak-linked deaths, as reported by the April 30th Weekly Epidemiology Report, based on the location where the infection occurred: either behind institutional walls defended by government, or out among the general population. From data shown in figure 8. Calculations in the Notes[1].

The little numbers on the pie chart are the actual raw numbers of outbreak-linked deaths in Canada as reported by the April 30th

Weekly Epidemiology Report. 13,611 deaths linked to infections caught on the government's side of the institutional divide. And only 178 deaths linked to infections on our side of the institutional barrier. **13,611 vs 178**. Those are the hard numbers illustrating the differences of what is occurring on either side of that institutional divide.

And don't worry, I will soon bring the other 10,613 deaths not linked to outbreaks into the story as this scandal continues to build. We'll climb this layer cake one layer at a time.

10 — Deflecting Blame: First Implications

When the numbers are sorted according to this institutional divide, the data becomes rather shocking. It doesn't matter what we do on the outside of this barrier. What matters is how well the government controls that barrier. It doesn't matter if every single school, church, shoe store, gym, restaurant, campground, nail salon, and meat packing plant in our country was bulldozed to the ground and vaporized by aliens with ray guns. The deaths on the inside of those institutions would continue, relentlessly, as long as the government fails to defend that barrier.

98.6% of the dying would continue, relentlessly, even if you arrested every single small business owner, pastor, worshipper, anti-lockdown protester, restauranteur, fitness enthusiast, anti-masker, nail salon owner, hair stylist, college student, party animal, and conspiracy theorist. You could lock us all in a stone quarry and throw away the key. You could increase social distancing to 90 feet. You could make everyone wear 10 masks. The collateral damage to those living outside those institutional walls would become even more extreme that it is already. But 98.6% of the dying would continue anyway as long as the virus continues to circulate inside these institutional walls.

Blaming those on the outside of that institutional barrier for the disaster happening inside is a convenient distraction that allows the government to try to escape accountability. By making the nuanced details of the epidemiological data so inaccessible to the general public, by refusing to have an honest debate with critics, and by labelling everyone who tries to raise a concern as a "conspiracy theorist", the government is deflecting from the fact that the government and not the general public is the one with marbles in its brain and blood on its hands. The longer this goes on, the greater the panic among the population, and the more extreme the desire becomes to control others using measures that fundamentally misunderstand the problem and, as you shall soon see, serve only to make the problem worse.

Now that we've taken a little pause to consider the first of the implications of what we've discovered so far, let's dive back into the data. Because now I am going to really blow your socks off. I am going to give you perspective on just how tiny that institutionalized population is and how badly fear is being blown out of proportion for those living outside of this institutional barrier. Put on your seatbelts because this is where magnitude of the scandal really becomes clear.

11 — Risks to the Elderly Living Inside vs Outside Institutional Settings

To expose the next layer of the scandal, I first need to take a small step backwards. The following chart is the age distribution of all 24,402 COVID-related deaths in Canada as of May 7th, 2021:

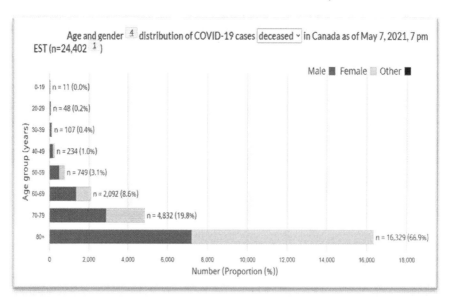

Figure 18: Age distribution of COVID deaths. Source: Canada's official daily epidemiological updates (Government of Canada, May 8, 2021).

You have probably seen the chart in figure 18 before. According to this chart, approximately 86.7% of all deaths in Canada are among people who are 70 and older. That rises to 95.3% if you include those between the ages of 60 and 69. It gives the impression that we are facing a pandemic that preys predominantly on the elderly. There is a kernel of truth to that statement, but only a very small kernel, because unless the age distribution data is combined with contact tracing details to identify the source of each fatal infection, this age distribution data creates a wildly distorted sense of risk.

According to Statistics Canada, there are approximately 9.4 million Canadians over the age of 60 (Statistics Canada, July 1st, 2020) living in Canada today. That's approximately 25% of the population. This demographic would appear, based on the impression created by Canada's age distribution graph, to be the demographic most at risk from the virus.

But let's go back to the outbreak data.

The outbreak data showed that 98.6% of all outbreak-related deaths are among cases caught inside institutional walls. And this is where any last remnants of doubt holding together the lockdown fantasy really come unglued.

Not all elderly with pre-existing conditions live inside institutional walls. Sounds obvious, right? But watch closely to what happens next as I put some numbers to the actual size of the high-risk populations living on either side of that institutional barrier.

- Long-term care residents: according to Census data there are approximately 160,000 people living in long-term care facilities in Canada (Hill Notes, October 22, 2020). Most (but not all) of those 160,000 long-term care patients are seniors (long-term care also has some younger residents with mental illness, handicaps, head injuries, and other severely debilitating conditions) but for the purpose of this exercise we can pretend they are all extremely vulnerable elderly.

- Hospital beds: there are approximately 95,000 hospital beds in Canada[2]. Clearly not all are filled with grievously ill seniors. There are also children's hospitals, maternity wards, ER wards, COVID treatment wards, and so on. And not every bed was full (in Ontario, hospital capacity rarely exceeded 90% at any time during this pandemic and even fell to historic lows (below 70% occupancy) during the first wave, although you may have gotten a different impression from statements of health officials and the scare stories promoted by the media. I have included a chart leaked form the Government of Ontario in the Notes[3] to illustrate this along with a chart from the UK, which demonstrates that low hospital utilization was not unique to our country[4]. I have also extensively documented the misrepresentation of overwhelmed hospitals in Canada during COVID an article on my website called *Bystander at the Switch: The Moral Case Against COVID Lockdowns.* (www.juliusruechel.com, January 29, 2021). So, although there are clearly far less than 95,000 seniors living as patients in hospitals in Canada, this number does put an upper bound on the *maximum* number of seniors that could be exposed to infection inside hospitals at any given time.

- Prisons: Canada has approximately 37,000 people (Statistics Canada, December 21, 2020) incarcerated across the country. Obviously only a small proportion are likely to be elderly, but again it puts an upper bound on the *maximum* number of law-breaking seniors that could be serving time in prison at any given time. That's good enough for where this story goes next.

That adds up to a maximum total of 292,000 potential seniors living inside these three institutional settings where 98.6% of the outbreak-linked deaths are occurring, versus at least 9.1 million seniors who live *outside* of this institutional barrier. A ratio of 1 to 31.

The following chart puts the size of these two elderly populations in context. The light-colored squares represent the *minimum* number of elderly living *outside* institutional walls. The dark-colored squares represent the *maximum* number of elderly living *inside* institutional walls where 98.6% of the outbreak-linked deaths happened.

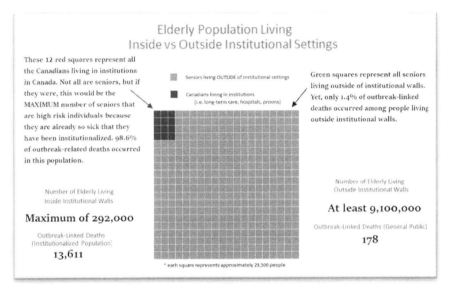

Elderly Population Living
Inside vs Outside Institutional Settings

These 12 red squares represent all the Canadians living in institutions in Canada. Not all are seniors, but if they were, this would be the MAXIMUM number of seniors that are high risk individuals because they are already so sick that they have been institutionalized. 98.6% of outbreak-related deaths occurred in this population.

Seniors living OUTSIDE of institutional settings

Canadians living in institutions
(i.e. long-term care, hospitals, prisons)

Green squares represent all seniors living outside of institutional walls. Yet, only 1.4% of outbreak-linked deaths occurred among people living outside institutional walls.

Number of Elderly Living
Inside Institutional Walls

Maximum of 292,000

Outbreak-Linked Deaths
(Institutionalized Population)
13,611

Number of Elderly Living
Outside Institutional Walls

At least 9,100,000

Outbreak-Linked Deaths (General Public)
178

* each square represents approximately 23,500 people

Figure 19: Seniors living outside of institutions (low-risk settings) vs the total institutionalized population in Canada (represents the maximum number of potential seniors living in high-risk settings). Our side of the institutional divide looks pretty safe. The government's side of the institutional divide is a disaster zone.

Imagine for a moment that every single outbreak-linked death had happened in one of these two elderly populations. That would mean 13,611 outbreak-linked deaths occurred among this tiny population of 292,000 elderly living on the *inside* of the institutional barrier account. Versus only 178 outbreak-linked deaths in a population of at least 9.1 *million* elderly living *outside* of the institutional barrier. Our side of the institutional divide looks pretty safe. The government's side of the institutional divide is a disaster zone.

It's important to point out that many of the elderly among those 9.1 million are every bit as sick and vulnerable as those living on the inside of that institutional barrier but are still living at home. Many are living with the same severe pre-existing conditions that exist inside long-term care homes:

- Stroke,
- Heart disease,
- Chronic lung disease,
- Cancer,
- Chronic obstructive pulmonary disease,
- Diabetes,
- Alzheimer's, Parkinson's, or dementia,
- Kidney disease requiring regular dialysis,
- Morbid obesity,
- People receiving palliative care at home,
- People living with HIV who take antiretrovirals to suppress their immune system,
- People like my own father, who is head injured and requires 24-hour home-based care and almost always ends up with severe live-threatening pneumonia when he catches a cold. If my mother did not make the huge effort to provide home-based care, he *would* be living inside one of these long-term care facilities. And he would be among their most vulnerable residents.

Let's try to put some numbers to how many elderly live outside of these institutions with high-risk pre-existing conditions.

Data from the USA on the number of people living with multiple chronic conditions allows us to guesstimate what kind of numbers we're talking about. Canadians are slightly healthier, but these numbers get us in the right ballpark.

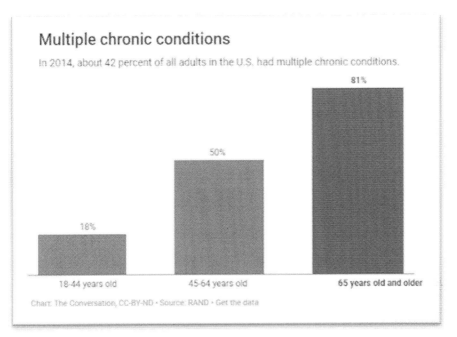

Figure 20: Percentage of Americans living with multiple pre-existing conditions (The Conversation, July 6, 2018).

So, let's redraw a new version of the chart shown in figure 19 by projecting the American percentages onto the Canadian population to identify what percentage of the 9.4 million people over the age of 60 are living with multiple chronic conditions in Canada today. Before I show the chart, here's the math:

- If 50% of people between the ages of 60 and 65, and 81% of people over 65 are living with multiple chronic conditions, we get the ballpark figure of **6.8 million Canadians over the age of 60 living with *multiple* chronic conditions**. A paper by the Canadian Institute of Health Information (CIHI, 2011) shows that 74% to 79% of Canadians over the age of 65 have at least one and 50% have at least 2 chronic conditions, but the paper does not include data on 60- to 65-year-olds. So, my guestimate using US numbers is not exact, but it get us in the right ballpark and allows us to understand how risk is divided between those living inside versus those living outside these institutions. Even if we generously pretend that all 292,000 residents inside these institutions are elderly with multiple chronic conditions, that still leaves over 6.5 million elderly Canadians with multiple chronic health conditions living outside of institutions. Yet, at most 178 outbreak-linked deaths can be attributed to this vast vulnerable population living outside of government-controlled walls.

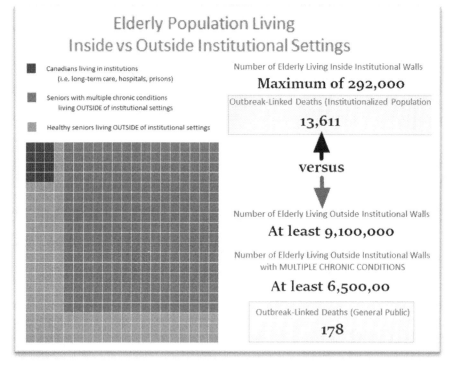

Figure 21: Seniors with *multiple chronic conditions* (medium grey) living outside of institutions (low-risk population), vs the total institutionalized population in Canada (black), which represents the maximum number of seniors living in high-risk settings. Light grey squares are the healthy seniors living without any pre-existing health conditions. Our side of the institutional divide *still* looks pretty safe, even for those with pre-existing conditions. The government's side of the institutional divide is still a disaster zone.

Yet the large population of vulnerable elderly Canadians with multiple pre-existing conditions who live outside of institutions (shown in medium grey in figure 21) are NOT dropping like flies. They are doing just fine. But God help those who are obliged to live under the government's care behind an institutional barrier (black squares in figure 21). You can probably guess by now where I'm going to take this investigation next...

How is it possible that almost all the deaths are stacked on one side of this institutional barrier but almost all the people (including the vast majority of those who are extremely vulnerable) are stacked on the other side?

The simple solution is that those on the outside have their own front door - their own defensive wall. Whereas those who rely on the government to defend them behind their institutional doors are being ravaged by this virus, seemingly without end, despite their tiny population. The tightest lockdown in the country, that of institutions, where every move made by every person inside can be controlled, is proving worthless despite being every Central Planner's dream come true. Yet everyday people that the government cannot control, but who are given information and retain the right to make their own choices about whether to leave their homes or bolt their front doors, are coming through this just fine.

A research paper published in the Lancet on March 17th, 2021 (Modiga et al., 2021) about the situation in Sweden came to the same conclusions: risk of death is much higher for those living in care homes, and pre-existing conditions are far more important than age. Here are a few quotes [my emphasis]:

"The results suggest that **age alone is not necessarily a risk factor for COVID-19-specific death, beyond the "normal" risk of age that is present in absence of the pandemic.**"

"Of special note was the relatively higher excess mortality among groups receiving care, suggesting that health status plays a more important role than age for COVID-19 associated deaths. Part of our findings may be

attributed to **differences in exposure to the virus between individuals receiving formal care and those living independently."**

If you have a little nagging doubt about the clear-cut story I've laid out so far, then you have been paying attention. Because there is an important loose end that needs to be tied up before I take you into those institutions to explain the scandal that has led to such a high death toll inside these institutions. This scandal goes way beyond our leaders presenting numbers without context and lying to conceal incompetence. It is a scandal of gross criminal negligence causing death. But to credibly reveal the crime, I first have to deal with the other 10,613 deaths that aren't accounted for by the outbreak data.

12 — Let's Bring in the Rest of the Data: ALL Deaths by Setting

Now that you understand this institutional barrier, which effectively divides Canada into two separate populations, it's time to bring in the rest of the data not included in the outbreak data set. Let's see how much the picture changes when ALL Canadian COVID deaths are held up against this institutional divide.

As I showed previously in figure 18, there were a total of 24,402 COVID deaths in the 15-month period ending May 7th, 2021. The outbreak data covered 13,789 of them, leaving 10,613 unaccounted for. It would be nice if the government provided the infection setting for those other 10,613 deaths, but it hasn't. Perhaps contact tracing wasn't possible for these infections. However, we do have some official data that allows us to allocate some of them, and we can give the government the benefit of the doubt for any that remain unaccounted for by putting the remainder on our side of the institutional barrier. Let's have a look at how the story changes:

Here's how I assigned the 10,613 deaths between the two sides of the institutional barrier:

- The Canadian Institute of Health Information has confirmed that 69% of all COVID deaths happened in just one setting (CBC News, March 30, 2021): long term care. Using that number, 69% of the 24,402 total deaths recorded on May 7th is 16,837 deaths in long-term care. Since 12,541 long-term care deaths are already accounted for by the outbreak data (figure 8), that adds another 4,296 deaths to the government's side of the ledger.

- If deaths not linked to outbreaks were happening at the same rate as outbreaks in each setting, we would have expected 9,647 (90.9%) of these 10,613 deaths to have occurred in long-term care. Instead, at 4,296, we only got 45% of that, which makes intuitive sense. Infections in closed institutional settings with vulnerable populations are easier to contact trace, so we would expect deaths not linked to outbreaks to be more common outside of institutional walls. So, we will use this same 45% number to guesstimate deaths linked to hospitals and prisons.

- The outbreak data (figure 8) showed that 1070 outbreak-linked deaths were linked to infections in hospitals and prisons (844 + 226). So, if the ratios from the outbreak data held true, 817 (7.7%) of the remaining 10,613 deaths would have occurred in hospitals and prisons, but again we'll reduce this to 45% of that amount to account for the fact that it is also easier to contact trace in hospitals and prisons. So, we'll add another 368 deaths to the government's side of the leger. This number is so small that it essentially doesn't matter which side of the ledger they go on in the context of the story.

- And that's it. That's as all the extra info we have. So, we'll give the government the benefit of the doubt and assign the balance - 5,949 deaths - to our side of the ledger (community spread).

Here's what the end result looks like:

Deaths linked to the source of infection

Inside institutional settings		Outside institutional settings	
Outbreaks (Long-term care, hospitals, prisons)	13,611	Outbreaks outside institutions	178
Long-term care, not linked to outbreaks	4,296	Balance of deaths	5,949
Hospitals & prisons, not linked to outbreaks	368	(give govt benefit of the doubt)	
	18,275		6127

Total 24,402

Figure 22: All COVID deaths in Canada, assigned by source of infections, giving the government the benefit of the doubt for any that we don't know the location of infection. **Yet, we still see 75% of all deaths occurring inside government institutions**.

These numbers make intuitive sense. But they also continue to expose the dramatic difference in death rates on either side of the institutional divide. **75% of <u>all</u> deaths are linked to infections in institutional settings**.

75% of all deaths are *among the tiny population of 292,000* living inside government-controlled institutions. Versus only 25% of all deaths spread out among the 38 million Canadians living outside of government institutions, including more than 6.5 million vulnerable elderly Canadians living with multiple chronic conditions!

Just to get a little extra visual perspective, let's recreate a similar chart to the ones shown in figures 19 and 21 to demonstrate the size of each of these populations on either side of the institutional barrier and how deaths are divided between these two separate worlds:

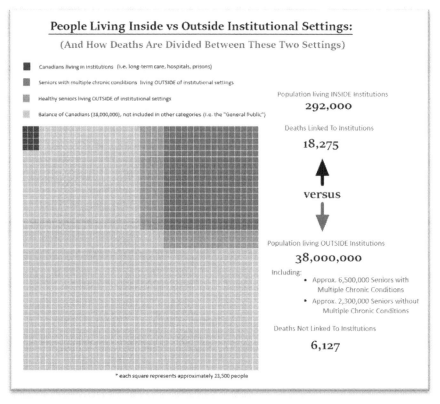

Figure 23: Population living inside institutional settings (black) versus everyone else (dark grey = seniors with multiple chronic health conditions, medium grey = healthy seniors, light grey = all other Canadians under the age of 60). And how deaths are divided between these two populations.

Since everyone prefers different types of charts to get perspective on a situation, here is another way to represent the data. I especially like this one:

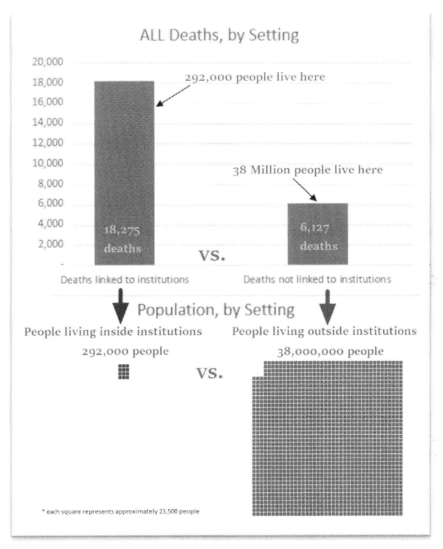

Figure 24: The government can't even protect the 292,000 people under its care. The public seems to be doing just fine by comparison.

It also is worthwhile to reflect back on the *14.5 million Canadians* who have travelled into Canada since the pandemic began. Travel didn't even warrant its own category in the outbreak data despite all the PCR testing and contact tracing that focused almost exclusively on travelers throughout the first wave of this pandemic. Yet the tiny population of only 292,000 people living inside institutions (1/50th the number of travelers) managed to rack up 75% of ALL deaths.

But the story is far from over. The scandal is about to take a darker turn. Now I'm going to show you why lockdowns are not just ineffective, but that they are responsible for many of the COVID deaths that have occurred among the vulnerable, quite possibly including the death of the infant in Dr. Henry's propaganda message at the beginning of this investigative report. The two separate but parallel populations living on either side of the institutional barrier are the key to unlocking the next layers of this scandal.

13 — Honest Numbers, Dishonest Health Officials, and a Blatant Disregard for the Rules

On January 29th, 2020, as health authorities first began to take notice of the virus spreading around the world, Canada's Chief Public Health Officer, Dr. Theresa Tam, warned that "*the epidemic of fear could be more difficult to control than the epidemic itself*" and that "*any measures that a country is to take must not be out of proportion to the risk.*" (HESA Committee Minutes, January 29, 2020) Dr. Tam correctly identified that the greatest risk of pandemic management is fear itself. Yet in the months that followed her warning turned into a prophesy, driven in no small part by her own public messaging.

The screenshot in figure 25 comes from the WHO's 2019 pandemic planning guide (WHO, 2019). It shows the different levels of health measures that a government can use to manage pandemics of various degrees of severity. The reason why these guidelines were created was not just to prevent panic-driven mistakes made in the heat of the moment, but just as importantly to *limit* government action in order to prevent sparking fear among the population. These guidelines are based on decades of research and on experiences gained from previous respiratory virus pandemics. Study this list carefully. Every limit placed on the government appears to have been ignored.

Table 1. Recommendations on the use of NPIs by severity level

SEVERITY	PANDEMIC*	EPIDEMIC
Any	Hand hygiene Respiratory etiquette Face masks for symptomatic individuals Surface and object cleaning Increased ventilation Isolation of sick individuals Travel advice	Hand hygiene Respiratory etiquette Face masks for symptomatic individuals Surface and object cleaning Increased ventilation Isolation of sick individuals Travel advice
Moderate	As above, plus Avoiding crowding	As above, plus Avoiding crowding
High	As above, plus Face masks for public School measures and closures	As above, plus Face masks for public School measures and closures
Extraordinary	As above, plus Workplace measures and closures Internal travel restrictions	As above, plus Workplace measures and closures
Not recommended in any circumstances	UV light Modifying humidity Contact tracing Quarantine of exposed individuals Entry and exit screening Border closure	UV light Modifying humidity Contact tracing Quarantine of exposed individuals Entry and exit screening Internal travel restrictions Border closure

NPI: non-pharmaceutical intervention; UV: ultraviolet.

Figure 25: Recommended public health measures suitable for pandemics of different severities. From the WHO's 2019 pandemic planning guide (WHO, 2019).

The measures used by the government during COVID are "off the chart." Contact tracing, quarantine of exposed individuals (i.e. health people who simply crossed paths with someone else who had the virus), entry screening at buildings and stores, and border closures are not to be used under ANY circumstances. Not only do these "off-the-chart" measures not work (i.e. experience shows that by the time you close the border, the virus is already circulating inside), they also heighten fear, which risks triggering panic in the population.

Based on the categories of the pandemic guidelines chart, the fact that government also used workplace closures, internal travel restrictions, and school closures would all suggest that we faced a pandemic of high or extraordinary severity. 24,402 deaths sound like a lot, right? You be the judge:

How severe was the COVID pandemic compared to previous years with normal mortality? The annual total of deaths (all causes) released by Statistics Canada allows us to compare the 2020 COVID year to previous years:

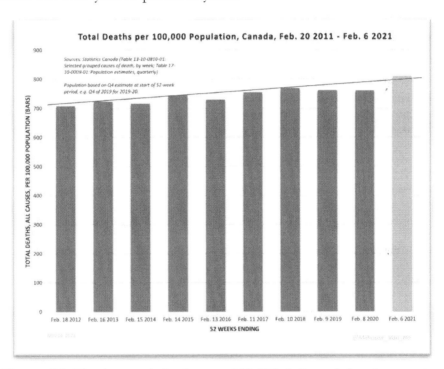

Figure 26: Total annual deaths per 100,000 (adjusted for the growing population size) from February of 2011 to February of 2021. The trendline laid across the top of the peaks illustrates the long-term growth in deaths attributed to an aging population. Extension above this trendline in 2021 illustrates the magnitude of the extra deaths during COVID beyond the peaks of previous bad flu seasons. Extra deaths are either caused by COVID or by the lockdown measures. (Adapted from @Milhouse_Van_Ho (Twitter, May 14, 2021) - the most accurate source tracking official Canadian government COVID data on the internet, found exclusively on Twitter with data sourced from Statistics Canada.)

The light grey column in figure 26 represents the first year with COVID and captures the first wave and almost the entire second wave (see figure 3 for reference). Yet it barely extends above the trendline laid out by previous bad flu seasons.

The other thing worth noting is that bad years are typically followed by mild ones. This is not necessarily a result of a more deadly strain of virus. The best analogy, however brutal it may be, is to compare it with the dry tinder that builds up in a forest, waiting for a spark. After a big fire, the forest becomes relatively fire-resistant until enough fresh tinder builds up again. In a flu season, the tinder is, sad to say, the population of vulnerable citizens, especially (but not exclusively) those living in long-term care facilities where it is particularly challenging to prevent the virus from spreading among residents if it gets inside. COVID comes on the heels of two milder flu seasons, which came after the deadly winter flu year of 2017/18 (I provide many examples in my article called *Bystander at the Switch: The Moral Case Against Lockdowns* (www.juliusruechel.com, January 25, 2021) demonstrating how badly hospitals were overflowing during the 2017/28 flu season). The virus is real, but it is far from a once-in-a-lifetime pandemic like the 1918 Spanish Flu.

These numbers may surprise you. 24,402 deaths represent approximately 8% of the total number of people that die in Canada every year (Statistics Canada, November 26, 2020). The light grey column in figure 26 is nowhere near an 8% bump over the numbers of previous years, even if you measure off the bottom of the 2019 trough. It is easiest to explain this strange phenomenon by looking at this statement in a recent article, made by BC's chief medical officer for the Interior BC region, Dr. Albert de Villiers:

As he's noted in the past, others who've contracted COVID-19 and died in long-term care homes may have shown no symptoms from the virus itself.

"This is a facility where there are people who are elderly, and have got some concurrent diseases as well, and some of the people who passed away were palliative before they got COVID," Dr. de Villiers said.

Figure 27: BC's chief medical officer for Interior BC, quoted by Castanet News article called *Half of deaths unvaccinated* in Kelowna, BC, on May 21st, 2021 (Castanet, May 21, 2021)

What Dr. Albert de Villiers is pointing out is that many COVID deaths are deaths *with* but not *from* COVID. These are people who died of other causes but also had a positive PCR test, even if they showed no symptoms from COVID itself. Including people already receiving palliative care — these are people who are dying of other causes, imminently, within days or weeks, and there is no longer anything that can be done to stop it.

Considering that 75% of all COVID deaths in Canada occurred inside government institutions, especially hospitals and long-term care, wouldn't it be nice if the government provided this context? By not making this distinction, it inflates the numbers. That may be useful for epidemiologists to track the spread of a virus, but it is grossly irresponsible and completely contrary to the fiduciary duty of our public health officials to withhold this context while educating the public about their risks.

Mass PCR testing has never been used before to test all nursing home patients for the presence of respiratory viruses, regardless of their underlying cause of death. It is a well-known phenomenon that the immune systems of people who are nearing the end of their lives are essentially in the process of shutting down. Dying is a process, not a one-day event. As their immune systems slowly shut down, they become increasingly susceptible to picking up all sorts of viruses. In many cases the presence of the virus is merely a side show to the actual cause of death. At most, it is the straw that breaks the camel's back. In many cases the presence of the virus found in a PCR test is as an inconsequential in the patient's death as the flowerpot standing in the corner of the room. If you did mass PCR testing of nursing home patients for all the other respiratory viruses that cause colds and flus (there are hundreds), you would find tons of them.

And if you decided to ignore all this context and started doing mass PCR testing for influenza virus in palliative care patients using the lax "case" definition used for COVID, and then gave the virus a fancy name and kept a running case count and death count on the front pages of newspapers, you would be able to create mass panic just like we have today, every single winter. This misuse of a diagnostic aid to do mass PCR testing of every patient and every death in long-term care facilities and hospitals is unethical, it is scientific fraud, and it is a criminal breach of trust in light of the illusion of mass dying that it creates.

Here's another official confirmation of this inflation of COVID deaths, straight from the official Twitter account of Toronto Public Health:

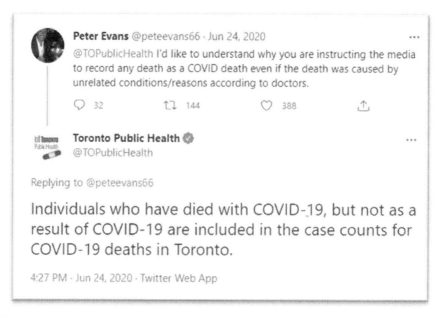

Figure 28: Toronto Public Health confirmed that case counts include deaths with COVID that were not necessarily caused by COVID (Twitter, June 24th, 2020).

Figure 29 uses Statistics Canada's own data to provide a clue of just how many "COVID" deaths may have been deaths *with* instead of *from* COVID. Look at the first three columns in particular - does COVID cure heart disease and cancer? It seems more likely that heart disease and cancer patients who would have died anyway were either misattributed to COVID as a result of a concurrent positive PCR test, as described by Dr. Albert de Villiers in the Castanet news article, or bad management of long-term care facilities unnecessarily exposed these already vulnerable individuals to the virus, thereby robbing them of the last few weeks or months of their life by pulling their death forward - the straw that broke the camel's back a few weeks or months early.

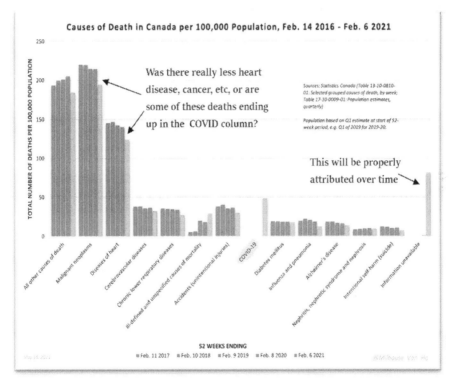

Figure 29: Causes of death during the first year of the pandemic. Adapted from @Milhouse_Van_Ho (Twitter, May 14, 2021), with data sourced form Statistics Canada.

It's not just the deaths of the elderly that are affected by this phenomenon. The Toronto Sun reported (Toronto Sun, May 21, 2021), according to the Public Health Agency of Canada only **36.6%** of children hospitalized with COVID were actually admitted with a COVID infection. In other words, a full *63.4% of children were admitted to hospital for treatment for other non-COVID health issues and caught COVID while they were on the inside of the hospital.* Hospital transmission, not community transmission. Just like the infant in Dr. Henry's propaganda masterpiece. Yet another quiet release of real information against a backdrop of noise about "cases, cases, cases" and rogue pastors to keep the public distracted and in the dark. The magician's tool of misdirection at its finest.

"Only 36.6% of pediatric patients hospitalized with COVID-19 were admitted due to an acute respiratory infection," explains a new report out from PHAC's Canadian Nosocomial Infection Surveillance Program (CNISP).

The report was quietly released last week. The term nosocomial refers to illnesses that originated within a hospital setting.

This means that out of the number of children previously tallied to have been in hospital with COVID-19, only a third of them were actually in hospital because they were in fact suffering from COVID-19, pneumonia or something similar.

Figure 30: *FUREY: Fewer Canadian kids hospitalized with COVID than previously thought, report shows*, (Toronto Sun, May 21st, 2021)

The next chart shows the running totals of weekly deaths (all causes) going back over the last 11 years, ending February 6th, 2021. The clear peaks and troughs in figure 31 represent **seasonal variations** in death rates caused by the winter flu season. Strong peaks correspond with especially strong winter flu seasons. The strong 2017/18 season is clearly visible.

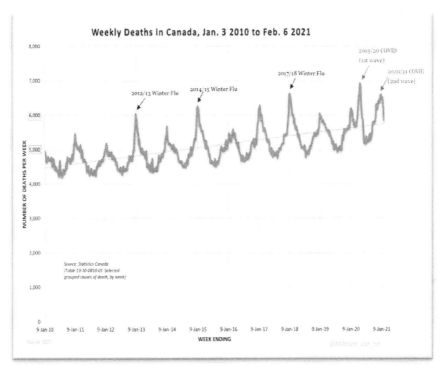

Figure 31: Causes of death during the first year of the pandemic. Adapted from @Milhouse_Van_Ho (Twitter, May 14, 2021), with data sourced form Statistics Canada.

The first two COVID waves of the 2019/20 and the 2020/21 winter seasons are recognizable on the chart in figure 31, *but do not stand out from the pack*. A glance to the left shows that there are between *5000 and 6000 deaths per week in Canada*, every single week of the year, of all causes. In 2019, that added up to a total of 284,082 (Statistics Canada, November 26, 2020). That's the background of normal mortality in Canada from *all* causes of death. The gradual rise in death rates over the last decade, which is visible in the chart, is caused by a combination of a growing population and an aging population as the large numbers of baby boomers begin to reach the top of the age pyramid and birthrates fall (I have included a diagram of the changing age pyramid from 1980 to 2020 in the Notes for those not familiar with how Canada is "aging out"[5]).

In figure 31, COVID stands out as a bad flu year, not as a generational pandemic. It looks virtually indistinguishable from previous bad flu years. Measuring from the centerline (dotted line) to the peaks, even the deadly 1st wave of COVID is approximately the same as the scale of the 2012/13, the 2014/15, and the 2017/18 winter flu peaks. And the second wave, when we spent the winter in near endless lockdowns, including curfews in Quebec, endless business closures, and the arrest of multiple pastors across Canada who refused to limit church attendance, that second wave barely counts as a moderate winter flu season. Overwhelmed hospitals were a complete lie (documented in my previous article (www.juliusruechel.com, January 25th, 2021)), not because some hospitals didn't reach near 100% capacity (some did), but because our hospitals reach and exceed 100% capacity *every year*. Hospital utilization during the first year and a half of the pandemic has been significantly lower than usual; for the first time in years no-one was practicing any hallway medicine in Canada. But cancer patients had their treatments cancelled and surgeries delayed. They may pay the ultimate price for the panic.

One of the "mysteries" of the COVID pandemic has been the disappearance of the winter flu. COVID is now playing the role that influenza used to play - flu deaths have been displaced by COVID deaths. The chart in figure 31 makes that rather obvious. And the insight we gained from the outbreak data, demonstrating that 75% of *all* deaths are in institutional environments, makes it quite clear that the most vulnerable to COVID are the very same vulnerable people, hanging out in the very same settings, which would have been at risk of severe outcomes from influenza. Anyone can catch a SARS-CoV-2 infection, but the Grim Reaper stalks the vulnerable. A coronavirus playing the role that influenza used to play.

Health authorities, including Dr. Tam herself (CTV News, March 31, 2021) have given the impression that the flu has disappeared because of the effectiveness of masks, social distancing, and lockdowns. That's rubbish. If masks and social distancing and lockdowns can keep other respiratory viruses at bay, why not COVID? The SARS-CoV-2 virus and the influenza virus are almost identical in size and are spread via virtually identical mechanisms. Health authorities are taking credit for a natural phenomenon called viral interference and displacement (Wu et al., 2020), where a dominant virus suppresses the activity of other viruses. This phenomenon was well-known (Schultz-Cherry, 2015) long before COVID, but they are exploiting the fact that the public doesn't know about this phenomenon to validate their health measures. You can learn more about viral interference and displacement in this article included in the references (Nickbakhsh et al., 2019).

Another natural phenomenon being used to lie about the supposed effectiveness of lockdowns is that of seasonality. The previous chart in figure 31 showed the natural rises and falls in deaths every winter. The magnitude may change, but the waves are as predictable as winter snow in Canada. Figure 32, from Ontario Public Health, shows the seasonality of the other coronaviruses (of which there are at least 4), which circulate in the community and in long-term care facilities every winter as part of cold and flu season. Just because most members of the public hadn't heard about coronaviruses before doesn't change that they have been around for a long time and a lot is known about them.

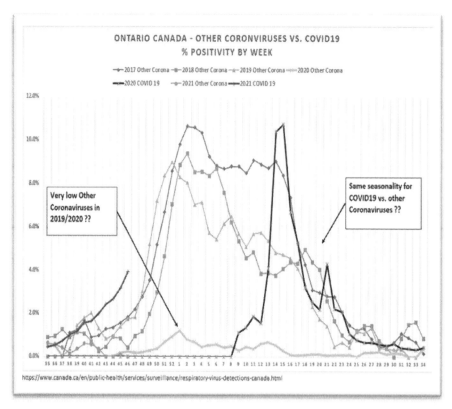

Figure 32: Normal seasonality of all coronaviruses in Canada. COVID-19 is merely the most recent addition. COVID arrived in Canada midway through the 2019/20 winter season (black line), and then tracked the other coronaviruses almost perfectly. And in the 2020/21 season (dark blue), it again appears to be tracking the other coronavirus waves from previous years. There are at least 4 other coronaviruses that have long been part of the regular annual smorgasbord of over 200 respiratory viruses that cause colds and flus every year (Government of Canada, June 3, 2021). Chart annotations are mine.

Bear in mind that the chart in figure 32 was published by our own health officials - they're even the ones who added the COVID numbers! Yet after every wave of COVID ends, health officials all around the world persist in taking credit for the natural seasonal downturn in virus activity - a natural and predictable seasonal phenomenon. It's like taking credit for the sun rising in the East.

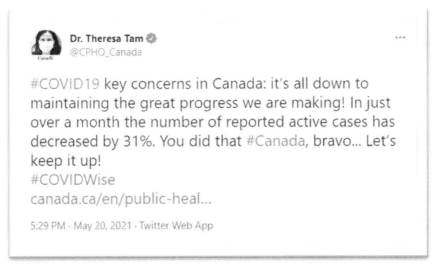

Dr. Theresa Tam ✓
@CPHO_Canada

#COVID19 key concerns in Canada: it's all down to maintaining the great progress we are making! In just over a month the number of reported active cases has decreased by 31%. You did that #Canada, bravo... Let's keep it up!
#COVIDWise
canada.ca/en/public-heal...

5:29 PM · May 20, 2021 · Twitter Web App

Figure 33: Dr. Theresa Tam, Chief Public Health Officer of Canada, giving public health measures (and compliance) credit for the natural seasonal variability of coronaviruses (Twitter, May 20, 2021).

No, Dr. Tam, we did not do that. Seasonality did.

A remarkable article published in the Telegraph on May 14th, 2021 (The Telegraph, May 14, 2021), reports that a group of scientists have admitted to using fear to control people's behavior during the COVID pandemic. Abir Ballan of *pandata.org*, an organization which has been compiling epidemiology data from around the world to provide the transparency that our governments have abandoned, reported on the article on Twitter. I encourage you to read Abir's full thread (Twitter, May 22, 2021) - it is eye-opening, to say the least.

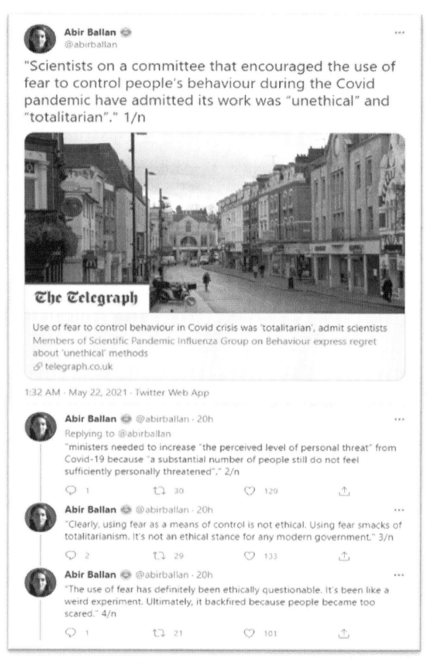

Figure 34: Partial thread by Abir Ballan on Twitter discussing the breaking story in the Telegraph of scientists admitting to using fear to control people's behavior. I encourage you to read her full thread (Twitter, May 22, 2021).

What these health officials and scientific advisory boards have done is not just shameless exploitation. It is scientific fraud, with real, serious, and deadly consequences for all those whose lives are being destroyed by lockdowns. This fear-driven public messaging reinforces the idea that if you want to save grandma, you must control the behavior of people living out in the community, outside of institutional walls. It reinforces the myth that lockdowns work. That lockdowns save lives. That masks and social distancing and well-behaved pastors and hairdressers are the key to keeping everyone safe.

This idea is not just false. This strategy is actually killing people. And I don't just mean deaths caused by collateral damage from lockdowns. I also mean COVID deaths themselves because lockdowns drag out the length of the pandemic, leading to thousands of unnecessary and entirely preventable deaths from COVID among the most vulnerable. Added together across the world, this could easily stretch into *millions of preventable COVID deaths* by the time this madness ends. This may sound like an extreme claim — let me walk you through it. We have reached the part of the story where their gross criminal negligence is laid bare in its rawest form.

14 — How Lockdowns Bring Death to the Vulnerable

The fantasy of lockdowns is that they flatten the curve:

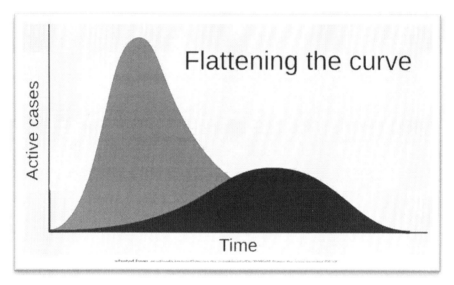

Figure 35: The fantasy behind flattening the curve.

This is just plain wrong. You saw the real-world data with your own eyes. Death from respiratory viruses follow a cyclical seasonal pattern. You can't stretch the season. You can only blunt the top of the peak by transferring infections to the next season. COVID, like all other coronaviruses and influenza, is seasonal.

We used lockdowns to slow the spread of the virus. We now have two whole winter seasons behind us but thanks to lockdowns slowing down the spread among the healthy and the least vulnerable, the community at large has still not achieved herd immunity. This means that the vulnerable are still trapped behind locked doors, either in institutions or at home. And they are still at risk of catching the virus from every single community member they encounter, 18 months in and no end in sight. *"Flatten the curve"* was just a noble-sounding euphemism for *"keep the vulnerable at risk for more than 18 months by preventing the community from building a protective ring of natural herd immunity around them."*

Yet if the government had followed the pandemic planning guidelines and provided focused protection for the vulnerable, while allowing the virus to spread among the rest of society as the winter flu does every winter, then the vulnerable would have been able to get back to their lives after 6 to 8 weeks of carefully guarding their doors.

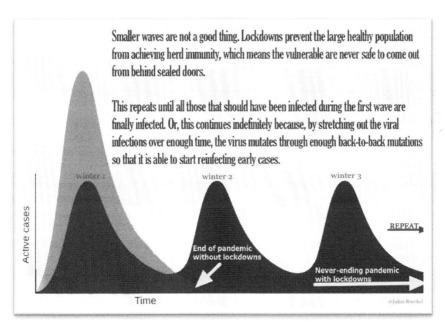

Figure 36: Lockdowns create wave after wave of smaller seasonal waves, thus condemning the vulnerable to be at permanent risk from the rest of society. The longer this process takes, the more of them will be exposed to the virus, despite the best efforts to keep the doors locked, thus *increasing* death among the vulnerable. Lockdowns mean the dying never ends

among the vulnerable because they remain at risk from the community around them.

Remember the chart in figure 3 (reproduced below) showing the waves of deaths in Canada? The second wave is extremely important to understand the impact of lockdowns:

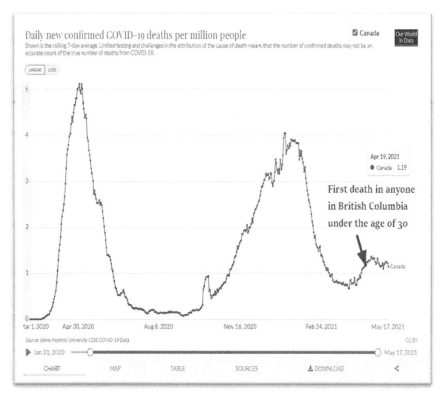

Figure 37: Canada's COVID waves (not much of a third wave either), showing the date of BC's first death of anyone under the age of 30. (World in Data, March 17, 2021)

As you know, the overwhelming majority of deaths occurred among the extremely vulnerable, particularly among those living in long-term care and among patients going to hospitals to seek treatment for other conditions, just like the infant in Dr. Henry's propaganda story. If the government had not imposed lockdowns, the majority of the broader community would have been exposed to and would have acquired natural immunity to the virus by the end of the first wave. Thus, there would have been very few symptomatic infections circulating in the broader community by the time this infant was admitted to the BC Children's Hospital. Which means there would also have been far fewer patients bringing the virus into the hospital and far less risk of this vulnerable infant getting exposed to it. *Without lockdowns, there may not have been a virus waiting to take down this infant by the time it arrived at the BC Children's Hospital 14 months after COVID arrived in Canada.*

The key to protecting the vulnerable is to dry up the virus outside. The gross negligence of abandoning pandemic planning guidelines has ensured that it is still there. Gross negligence may be the reason why this infant's death was entirely preventable. It most certainly caused the death of countless others because public health officials used lockdowns to create conditions to sustain a pandemic without end. A very large portion of the second wave of deaths (and beyond) were entirely preventable if the vulnerable living inside institutions had been given focused protection during the first wave while the virus was allowed to circulate freely outside among the community. In other words, much of the second wave of dying was preventable if the pandemic planning guidelines had not been ignored. DIY pandemic management means these health officials and politicians have *millions* of deaths on their consciences. And they will need to answer for them in a court of law once the hysteria subsides.

And it doesn't stop there. The number of vulnerable citizens is not a fixed population. Even as some gain immunity and others die of natural causes, their numbers are constantly being replenished with newcomers who join the ranks of the vulnerable. If the virus had been allowed to circulate freely in the community without lockdowns (focused protection only), there would only have been a 6 to 8 week period during which the vulnerable would have needed focused protection (bolted doors), but *by extending this period over a year and a half, thousands of people who were not vulnerable during the 1st wave now been added to the ranks of the vulnerable,* perhaps because they became ill with cancer, or leukemia, or heart disease.

And, because many of these once healthy but now sick individuals did not acquire herd immunity while they were still healthy during the first wave, they do not bring any immunity with them to long-term care homes and hospitals and do not have the necessary immunity to fight off COVID if they catch it now that they are weak. *By denying them the chance to get exposed to the virus while they were strong, they now face a significantly higher risk of death if they are exposed to it while they are weak.*

For example, the infant in the Dr. Henry's propaganda story may or may not have already had pre-existing conditions during the first wave. Perhaps it only developed these vulnerabilities after the second wave. Had the virus been allowed to circulate freely in the community during the first wave, there would have been a lot lower risk of the virus being present in the hospital when the infant arrived for treatment. And perhaps, if schools and daycares and workplaces had not been shuttered during the first wave, the infant may already have acquired immunity to the virus during the first wave, which would have prevented it from dying when it caught COVID after arriving at the BC Children's Hospital.

And consider long-term care home populations. This article from the US (UCSF, 2010) shows that the average length of stay in a long-term care facility before death is 13.7 months, while the median length of stay is only 5 months. This means that *half of all long-term care residents live less than 5 months in long-term care.* They don't have time for a year-long lockdown. Three separate "crops" of long-term care patients have come and gone since COVID began. And yet there is still no safety to be found inside these institutions because the virus still hasn't been allowed to burn itself out outside.

Lockdowns have stretched out the isolation so long that many of these patients have been robbed of the last precious months with family members and were left to face death in isolation, without the dignity and comfort of being surrounded by loved ones during their most difficult moments. It breaks my heart. Some, like Nancy

Russell (CTV News, November 19, 2020), chose assisted suicide rather than face the isolation of another lockdown.

And yet our health officials had the all the information needed to prevent this from happening and demonstrated knowledge of those pandemic planning guidelines before they abandoned them.

> ## Guarantee of Rights and Freedoms
> ▬▬▬ 1. The *Canadian Charter of Rights and Freedoms* guarantees the rights and freedoms set out in it subject only to such reasonable limits prescribed by law as can be demonstrably justified in a free and democratic society.

Figure 38: Section 1 of the Canadian Charter of Rights and Freedoms

And they didn't just ignore guidelines. They systematically and knowingly violated our Charter of Rights and Freedoms, which is meant to act as the ultimate buffer against this kind of DIY rulemaking. Section 1 of the Charter places the burden of proof on the government to justify *any* limits put on our rights and freedoms - in a court of law - *before* it has the right to impose those limits. I have reproduced Section 1 of our Charter for you in Figure 38. *It is an obligation placed on government to provide the burden of proof before it can limit our rights and freedoms. Section 1 gives us our right to demand transparency and public debate.* It specifically denies government the arbitrary right to decide when some "greater good" is sufficiently important for government to unilaterally suspend our rights and freedoms.

Thanks to these inalienable individual rights, health orders can only be recommendations, not mandatory orders, unless they pass the burden of proof (in a court of law) as required by Section 1 of our Charter. Thus, even if health officials and politicians were too incompetent or too uninformed to follow the pandemic planning guidelines, all they should have been able to do is make stupid and ill-advised recommendations. Our constitutional rights should have prevented them from imposing mandatory lockdowns and other measures to "flatten the curve", which have dragged out this pandemic for more than a year and a half and counting. It would have eliminated the government's ability to control the community, yet everyone would have retained the right to bolt their own doors (and therefore take responsibility for their own safety while the virus raged outside). And the government would still have had the exact same tools available to them to provide focused protection to the vulnerable living inside institutions.

The legal process required for the government to pass this burden of proof to limit our constitutional rights in Canada is called the Oakes Test (Center for Constitutional Studies, n.d.). It is meant to force politicians, health officials, and scientists through a gauntlet of debate and evidence-based discussion and stop them from engaging in ad-hoc rulemaking. *This never happened.* And because every other country is doing it too, it normalized the idea that our inalienable individual rights have been downgraded to conditional individual rights. But they are not. In the United States, their constitution doesn't even have a provision for suspending inalienable. Yet they did it too, irregardless.

Lockdowns are an experiment that has never been done before. A type of medieval medical experiment involving *billions* of lives, without a shred of evidence to support it, despite clear guidelines not to do it, and despite human rights meant to prevent it. Lockdowns are illegal. Every single health official and politician that imposed them *must* stand trial for *human rights violations* once the panic subsides and people come to their senses, because that is the legal term for when mass violations of human rights occur and when large numbers of deaths happen as a result.

Sadly, that is not the only thing they will have to answer for in a court of law. The game they have been playing to use fear to control people's behavior has also had lethal consequences, on top of those already caused by lockdowns. That's the next chapter of this scandal. And as usual, it is the vulnerable inside institutions who are paying the price, with their lives, for the direct consequences of the panic that was intentionally provoked by our government.

15 — The Price of Fear

Yelling "fire" in a crowded theatre is illegal. The fear whipped up by health care officials, politicians, and media during COVID is the medical equivalent of this crime. Fear combined with a disregard for our constitutional rights and freedoms produced an especially toxic and deadly combination. It focused the full force of human creativity on a singular mission to control other people "for safety" in a hysterical "anything goes" free-for-all that was released from the limiting restraints provided by individual rights, unshackled from the brakes of democratic norms, and exempt from the need to provide transparent evidence and engage in debate, which are essential for science to function properly.

I shall begin with the fear caused by face masks, whose effectiveness has no demonstrable basis in science, but which have served to create a constant visual reminder of danger and heighten the public's sense of fear. The consequences of relying on face masks, and the fear that was unleashed by them, play a huge role in explaining why the tiny population of only 292,000 citizens living in institutions suffered more than 75% of *all* deaths in Canada.

Here's what the WHO has to say about face masks in their 2019 pandemic planning guidelines:

> **OVERALL RESULT OF EVIDENCE ON FACE MASKS**
>
> 1. Ten RCTs were included in the meta-analysis, and there was no evidence that face masks are effective in reducing transmission of laboratory-confirmed influenza.

Figure 39: Randomized controlled trials are the gold standard to test if a measure works. It was well-known before COVID that face masks have no effect on the spread of respiratory viruses (WHO's 2019 pandemic planning guidelines).

I have previously written a deep dive, called *Droplets and Aerosols: Why Catching the Sneeze Doesn't Reduce Viral Transmission*, published on my website (www.juliusruechel.com, September 29, 2020), about the scientific explanation for why face masks don't work and the consequences of trying to protect the vulnerable with what ultimately amounts to a placebo. I will briefly summarize the key takeaways relevant to the discussion in this investigative report. The study of droplets and aerosols shows that coughing and sneezing produces droplets that are predominantly larger than 5 microns in diameter (the virus itself is around 0.12 microns in diameter). Any droplet larger than 5 microns will quickly settle out of the air because of gravity. So, unless a drop settles on your finger and then you pick your nose, it is difficult to introduce these droplets into your respiratory system. That's why hand washing works.

But regular breathing produces aerosols of around 0.07 microns and congested breathing (i.e. from *symptomatic* people) produces aerosols of 0.2 to 0.5 microns. These are small enough to stay suspended in the air for a long time, to get sucked through ventilation ductwork, to get inhaled, and to go through N95 masks and HEPA filters. N95 masks and HEPA filters only reliably catch particles down to 0.3 microns in size, so they mostly catch what gravity solves anyway. A 0.12-micron virus inside a 0.2-micron aerosol passes right through all these masks. This knowledge about aerosol sizes explains the results of the randomized controlled studies. Masks are pointless for stopping respiratory viruses, even though they are useful for larger particles like bacteria, dust, and pollen.

In the early days of the pandemic, every single health authority all around the world told us that face masks don't work and that we should not wear them. They were correct. This message in the early days of the pandemic demonstrates a clear knowledge of the WHO pandemic planning guidelines and the established science on masks:

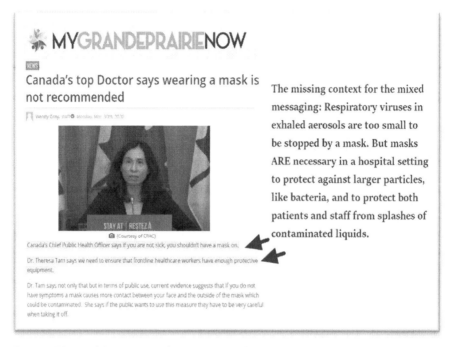

The missing context for the mixed messaging: Respiratory viruses in exhaled aerosols are too small to be stopped by a mask. But masks ARE necessary in a hospital setting to protect against larger particles, like bacteria, and to protect both patients and staff from splashes of contaminated liquids.

Figure 40: Dr Tam (Canada's Chief Public Health Officer of Canada) in the news: mixed messaging ignited fear among the public. Dr. Tam was right in both statements, but without context it unleashed unbridled panic (My Grande Prairie Now, March 20, 2020).

Health authorities also told the public that frontline healthcare workers *do* need them (also correct), but without telling them why (to protect against bacteria and to protect health care workers from splashes of contaminated liquids (i.e., cough splatter, urine, etc.) while on the job). Because the context for why health care workers and long-term care staff *do* need masks was so poorly communicated, it created a mixed message that gave the public the impression that the government was downplaying the risks.

The government didn't fix its inept wording to explain the nuanced details between these seemingly contradictory messages. Fear increased and mask shortages increased. Care home staff were left short and scared because they felt unprotected. Many staff members fled, leading to countless horrifying examples (Montreal Gazette, April 8, 2020) of unnecessary care home deaths around the world among patients who were abandoned in their beds. The analogy of yelling fire in a crowded theater is remarkably apt.

At this point it was obvious that the public had latched onto a false idea of safety and was winding itself into a knot of fear. But instead of recognizing what was happening and working to try to allay those fears, the government capitulated to those fears and gave the public (or at least the noisy voices in click-hungry media) what it wanted - a mask recommendation - thereby reinforcing the sense of danger with a permanent visible symbol that reminds everyone that everyone else is to be feared.

They made this switch without offering a single new randomized controlled study - it was pure theory pulled out of thin air. (In my article called *Opinion is Not Evidence, Ignoring Science to Follow Gut Instinct* (www.juliusruechel.com, September 29, 2020) I documented the source of the sudden about-face on masks: it was a decision based on political lobbying, not science). Now, instead of just fearing those who cough, sneeze, and wheeze, fear increased to include everyone who breathed.

This started the snowball rolling towards mandatory mask laws, mandatory social distancing, PCR testing of asymptomatic people, and mandatory lockdowns because once everyone was wearing a mask, everyone looks dangerous. And if everyone is dangerous, then everyone's survival depends on controlling the movements and even the breathing of others.

Fear is not rational. That is why public health officials must work so hard to *prevent* it. They must never give in to impulses that promote it, much less use it as a tool to shape behavior, because these forces are not controllable once they are unleashed. And the unintended consequences are deadly.

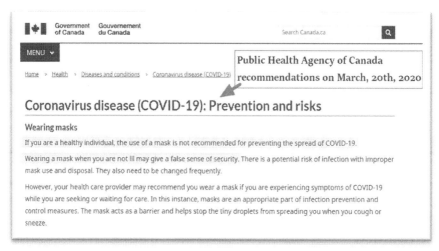

Figure 41: The Public Health Agency of Canada's stance on masks in March of 2020. "*Wearing a mask when you are not ill may give a false sense of security.*" (Government of Canada, March 20, 2020)

The first of these unintended deadly consequences is that masks provide a false sense of security for those who *are* vulnerable. While most of us should have carried on living our lives, as blissfully unaware as possible, those who are vulnerable should be educated to keep a heavy door between themselves and the rest of society while the viral wave passes. But a mask gives a false sense of security, encouraging those who are vulnerable to mingle when mingling poses a mortal risk. Real world outbreaks like the outbreak at Tönnies meat packing plant in Germany (Swiss Policy Research, date) showed that a symptomatic worker infected co-workers as far as 26 feet away despite everyone in the facility *wearing a mask, including the symptomatic spreader*. So much for social distancing. So much for masks.

Asymptomatic people will have little or no virus particles inside the aerosols they exhale. But the aerosols exhaled by symptomatic people will be saturated with virus particles. The big drops that are expelled by coughs and sneezes quickly end up on the floor. But the tiny particles exhaled during normal congested breathing will be floating around the room and get sucked through heating ducts, just as they did on the *Diamond Princess* cruise ship (Wikipedia, 2020)

If the vulnerable go into a room with other masked individuals, they will not be protected against virus-containing aerosols expelled by breathing. How many vulnerable people living outside of government institutions died because of the false sense of security provided by masks? While the rest of us should have been mingling, they should have been getting their groceries delivered to the door. But why worry, they had masks to protect them, right?

But the biggest sin was what happened inside long-term care homes. Again, the endless list of catastrophes just don't end for nursing home residents. The government appears to have believed its own bullshit mask recommendations. Who needs science-based policies when you have a recommendation from someone with fancy credentials and a lab coat?

The default attitude when randomized controlled trials don't show any evidence of a mask working is to create policies *that err on the side of them not working*, not to assume that they do. The default is to trust the pandemic planning guidelines, not a political recommendation used to pander to a frightened public. But instead of focusing on ventilation to exhaust contaminated air and adopting strategies to divide residents into separate air spaces *without ventilation ducts connecting them* in order to minimize the mixing of aerosols between patients, masks and air filtration took the lead with their false promise to protect staff and residents from infection.

Up to 44% of deaths could have been prevented by eliminating staff cross-traffic (McKnight's Long-Term Care News, July 26, 2020) between nursing homes. But why worry, there's little risk if staff and residents are protected by masks, right?

Asking staff to live inside nursing homes with residents while doors remained sealed shut is a proven effective strategy to protect the vulnerable (McKnight's Long-Term Care News, August 18,

2020) while the viral wave passes outside. Few nursing homes used it. Everyone's wearing a mask, so why worry, right?

The experience of the COVID outbreak on the *Diamond Princess* cruise ship in February of 2020 showed rather clearly, long before COVID arrived in Canada, that the virus could spread effectively through ventilation ductwork. But why worry if masks and air filters work, right? Why trust real world experience, as shown by the Diamond Princess example, when you have a lab coat-endorsed recommendation?

An article published by *Aerosol and Air Quality Research* (Almilaji, 2020) discussed the spread through the ventilation system on the Diamond Princess. Princes Cruises *"confirmed that the HVAC filtration system on the Diamond Princess ship is comparable to those used by land-based hotels, resorts and casinos".* The authors go on to explain that *"HVAC systems in commercial setting have a minimum efficiency reporting value (MERV) of 5–8, in which MERV refer to the effectiveness of air filters in HVAC. And even in superior residential, commercial, and industrial spaces HVAC systems usually have a minimum efficiency reporting value (MERV) of 9–12."*

Isolating mask-wearing long-term care residents in their rooms achieved little as long as there was ductwork throughout the building. They might as well have been living on the Diamond Princess cruise ship. Even a HEPA filter is not much different than a mask - aerosols might not be able to go around a filter like they can around a mask, but they can still pass straight through. A 0.12-micron virus particle inside a 0.2-micron aerosol fits through 0.3-micron hole as easily as a mosquito fits through a chain-link fence. The default assumption based on both real-world experience and all the randomized controlled trials should have been that ducts and air filtration are not the solution to protecting the vulnerable in hospitals and long-term care facilities. Opening windows would have achieved far more.

And no, electrostatic forces are NOT a solution to stopping a virus with a HEPA filter, despite all the media hype. Here are a couple of quotes from a research article published by the National

Center for Biotechnology Information (Mousavi et al. 2020), which sums up the issue better than I can (emphasis mine):

"While US hospital construction standards require a minimum of MERV 13 or MERV 14 filtration for both fresh and recirculated air, **this level of filtration is not capable of reliably removing viral particles**" *[author's note: HEPA grade filters start at a MERV rating of 13]*

"The Centers for Disease Control and Prevention (CDC) recommends that hospitalized persons be placed in a single person room with the door kept closed, and **that an airborne infection isolation room (AIIR), also known as a negative pressure room, be used for such patients who may require an aerosol generating procedure in an effort to contain potentially infectious aerosols from patients known or suspected of an active infection due to SARS-CoV-2.**"

"Beyond acute care hospitals, nursing facilities typically have little to no capacity to provide an AIIR for patients. Instead, nursing facilities tend to transfer patients suspected of an infectious disease transmitted by small particle aerosols to a hospital for care and isolation in an AIIR for the duration of the period the patient may be contagious."

The inability of air filtration to stop virus particles *is a known fact in hospital construction.* They *know* electrostatic forces are not able to reliably overcome the size differential between a 0.2-micron aerosol and a 0.3-micron hole. Virus containment requires a negative pressure room to stop the spread *despite HEPA filtration.* Thus, the default position is to build policies around long-established research that filtration is not "capable of reliably removing viral particles" and NOT to suddenly believe they work.

Even the filter manufacturers are very careful to avoid making definitive legal claims that their filters are able to do anything reliably below the 0.3-micron range, despite glowing discussions about electrostatic forces being able to attract *some* smaller particles. These marketing claims are not backed up with hard numbers about any particle sizes being reliably stopped below 0.3 microns, much less what percentage of the sub-0.3-micron particles are trapped by these electrostatic forces. It is also well-known that chemical aerosols are able to pass straight through, despite also being below 0.3 microns - these tiny chemical aerosols need activated carbon filters to stop them so it would be very bizarre is similarly small virus-containing aerosols would follow different physical laws. Electrostatic forces are extremely weak forces.

Here are two quotes taking from the Vaniman website (Vaniman, March 20, 2020), a manufacturer of HEPA filters, about the ability to filter viruses with HEPA filters:

> *"The sad truth is that some viruses will inevitably pass through any HEPA filter."*

> *"Overtime, with enough volume or use, particles will eventually separate and penetrate the filter due to their sub-micron size."*

Yet despite everything that the health care industry knows about viruses, negative pressure rooms, and the limitations of air filtration, health officials nonetheless convinced themselves that it would be a good idea to transfer COVID-19 infected patients from hospitals into long-term care wards in order to free up hospital beds (The Globe and Mail, April 22, 2021). If anything, transfers should have been going in the opposite direction to get infected patients out of long-term care before they infect the other vulnerable residents. But hey, everyone's wearing masks and there's air filtration in the ducts. No problem, right?

And this deadly practice didn't just happen once. Even New York's disaster didn't stop the practice. Ontario was still transferring other hospital patients into long term care to free up beds in late April of 2021, *after 15 months of evidence stacking up to show how dangerous this practice is*!?! All it takes is one infected patient to introduce the virus into the entire building.

While they were gambling with the lives of the nursing home residents, they were lecturing us about delaying haircuts. Those stupid naughty plebs, why won't they listen to their enlightened lab coats? Children, don't even think about going to see your friends, you might kill grandma! All that collateral damage... if only pastors wouldn't open their churches so we could reach COVID-Zero! Some lessons are never learned because hubris gets in the way. The scale of our health officials' incompetence is staggering.

Meanwhile, many hotels stood empty, with tourism essentially on hold. Why weren't these used to make sure the hospital patients were kept as far away as possible from the vulnerable inside long term care facilities? Instead, hotels are now being used to quarantine the healthy when they come over the border, in direct violation of the pandemic planning guidelines and of our constitutional rights.

How many extra lives have been lost in Canada due to these horrific decisions and as a result of the horrific fear mongering? I don't know. Many. The dying hasn't stopped. The next wave has already begun. All because lockdowns have ensured that there still isn't enough herd immunity among the healthy low-risk members of the community to protect the vulnerable. But that's where the vaccine comes in, right? That's where we're going next in this scandal of endless preventable dying. Another sacred cow is on its way to slaughter...

I am left to wonder if we subtracted all the preventable COVID deaths from the totals, along with all the misattributed deaths, how many would be left? Would this pandemic stand out as anything unusual next to all the previous flu seasons? The healthy would not have died in larger numbers without lockdowns. But the vulnerable would have died in far fewer numbers without lockdowns. The epidemiological data and the lessons learned from the outbreak data set makes that quite clear - those at risk of death are a very specific vulnerable population. The more perspective we get, the clearer it becomes that this was largely a wave of dying caused by gross negligence on the part of the government.

The collateral damage caused by panic and by stretching this out over a year and a half (and counting) has been enormous. If life had carried on as per the WHO pandemic planning guidelines, life would have gotten back to normal about 15 months ago, with far fewer deaths.

And the collateral damage caused by the lockdowns in the community are spiraling. The Children's Hospital of Eastern Ontario is overwhelmed by so many children with mental health crises (caused by lockdowns) that it is on the verge of transferring patients to adult hospitals (CBC, April 18, 2021). Overdose deaths are soaring (Statistics Canada, March 10, 2020). Hundreds of thousands of medical treatments, surgeries, and diagnostic tests for serious high-risk high-mortality diseases, like cancer, were delayed or cancelled (Terrace Standard, February 7, 2021) all around the country, priming us for a future wave of additional unnecessary deaths because these patients didn't get the care they needed in the early stages of their diseases. And millions around the world have been pushed into poverty and starvation (World Food Programme, September 17, 2020) All these lives matter too. Pinning our hopes on vaccines as an exit strategy has been exceedingly costly, a price paid in many many lives.

16 — The Opportunity Cost of Waiting for a Vaccine and Ignoring Pandemic Planning Guidelines

The government and much of the public have embraced vaccination as the exit strategy for this crisis.

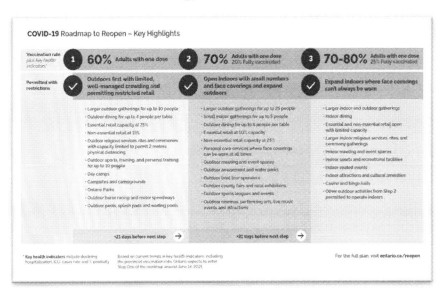

Figure 42: Government of Ontario reopening plan in May of 2021. By September of 2021, they had increased their vacation goal to 90%. The target keeps moving and the reopening never comes (Government of Ontario, June 9, 2021).

The logistical problems of rolling out a vaccine were inevitable. It was clear from the start that it would take more than a year to develop, manufacture and distribute a vaccine, perhaps longer. It was a gamble without a guarantee of achieving a safe or effective vaccine. And despite the rollout being underway, there are still no long-term safety trials (obviously), since they are still ongoing; they finish in 2024 (US National Library of Medicine, February 18, 2021). That is why these vaccines required emergency use authorization. We are the long-term trial.

Coercion is being used to force compliance, which is a violation under the Nuremberg Code (British Medical Journal, December 7, 1996) *(Full text of the Nuremberg Code (1947)* available in the notes at the bottom of this investigative report[6]). And we are on the cusp of introducing vaccine passports - a Chinese-style social credit score system for government-approved behavior, promoted under the guise of "safety" and introduced as a precondition to participating in normal life. It's Orwellian in the extreme.

But neither the 12+ month delay of waiting under lockdown for vaccines to arrive, nor the gamble about their safety, nor the threat to our civil liberties were ever necessary if we had just followed the pandemic planning guidelines. Vaccination increased deaths even before they arrived because, by pinning our hopes on them, we suffered through 18 months of lockdowns and an additional second wave instead of going through a single 6-to-8-week wave with focused protection for the vulnerable, as we would every year for a normal winter flu. It may be the deadliest vaccine in history not because of the vaccine itself but because of the terrible cost of maintaining endless lockdowns while we waited for them to arrive.

The alleged benefits of the vaccine are being sold as being a comparison between COVID deaths vs deaths caused by the vaccine. It is a false comparison. The real comparison is to compare the number of deaths caused by COVID if the pandemic guidelines had been followed versus all the extra deaths caused by lockdowns, flattening the curve, collateral damage, *plus* vaccine side effects. The real comparison is between all the time (and deaths) caused by waiting for a vaccine (plus its side effects) versus ripping off the band-aid as fast as possible by continuing to live a normal life while providing focused protection for the vulnerable. That is the real side-by-side choice that our health officials and politicians made for us.

So, the horror of looking to vaccines as an exit strategy from this crisis is that the false hope they created for a risk-free exit held the vulnerable hostage inside their homes and institutions, at risk from every member of the community they encounter, for over 18 months and counting. By pinning our hopes on the horizon, we prevented a ring of natural immunity from forming around the pockets of vulnerable. All because pandemic planning guidelines were ignored. All because everyone else in the community was prevented from living their lives. All because those with essentially zero risk from this virus were whipped into such a state of hysteria that they became afraid to live their lives without getting a jab. And now that they have one, they don't feel safe until everyone else gets one too.

17 — Is Informed Consent Even Possible for Those Who Have Natural Immunity? Implications of the Nuremberg Code.

And now that vaccines are here, guess who is bearing the brunt of the majority of adverse side effects? The vulnerable of course. The majority of injuries, permanent disabilities, and deaths are among the elderly, although there are also many young and middle-aged people with no history of pre-existing conditions who have also been injured or died. Dig into the case reports on VAERS (the Vaccine Adverse Event Reporting System maintained by the US CDC) - the case reports are eye opening and do not make for pleasant reading.

By mid-May, the US was approximately halfway to its vaccination goals; here are where their injuries and deaths linked to vaccination stood by that time:

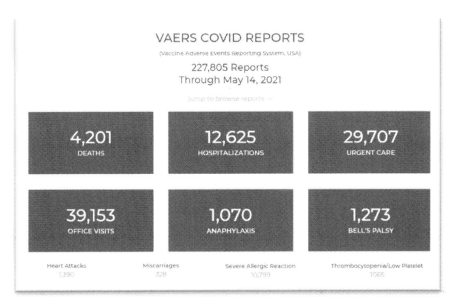

Figure 43: Summary of VAERS COVID reports (the Vaccine Adverse Events Reporting System maintained by the US CDC - US data only). Every country has its own system. This data only covers vaccinations performed in the United States. (OpenVAERS, May 14, 2021)

Messages:
▸ VAERS data in CDC WONDER are updated every Friday. Hence, results for the same query can change from week to week.
▸ These results are for 4,201 total events.
▸ Rows with zero Events Reported are hidden. Use Quick Options above to show zero rows.

Age ⬇	➡ Events Reported ⬆⬇	⬅ Percent (of 4,201) ⬆⬇
< 6 months	1	0.02%
1-2 years	3	0.07%
6-17 years	6	0.14%
18-29 years	37	0.88%
30-39 years	71	1.69%
40-49 years	130	3.09%
50-59 years	292	6.95%
60-64 years	287	6.83%
65+ years	2,983	71.01%
Unknown	391	9.31%
Total	4,201	100.00%

Elderly bearing the brunt

Note: Submitting a report to VAERS does not mean that healthcare personnel or the vaccine caused or contributed to the adverse event (possible side effect).

Query Criteria:

Event Category: Death
Vaccine Products: COVID19 VACCINE (COVID19)

Figure 44: VAERS Search: COVID Vaccine Deaths (VAERS, May 14, 2021)

Event Category ⬇	➡ Events Reported ⬆⬇	➡ Percent (of 227,805) ⬆⬇
Messages:		
▸ VAERS data in CDC WONDER are updated every Friday. Hence, results for the same query can change from week to week.		
▸ These results are for 227,805 total events.		
Death	4,201	1.84%
Life Threatening	3,868	1.70%
Permanent Disability	2,719	1.19%
Congenital Anomaly / Birth Defect *	121	0.05%
Hospitalized	12,625	5.54%
Existing Hospitalization Prolonged	164	0.07%
Emergency Room / Office Visit **	39	0.02%
Emergency Room *	29,669	13.02%
Office Visit *	39,151	17.19%
None of the above	156,624	68.75%
Total	**249,181**	**109.38%**

Note: Submitting a report to VAERS does not mean that healthcare personnel or the vaccine caused or contributed to the adverse event (possible side effect).

* These values are only available from VAERS 2.0 Report Form, active 06/30/2017 to present.
** These value are only available from VAERS-1 Report Form, active 07/01/1990 to 06/29/2017.

Query Criteria:

Vaccine Products: COVID19 VACCINE (COVID19)
Group By: Event Category

Figure 45: VAERS Search: COVID Vaccine Deaths (VAERS, May 14, 2021)

Over 4200 deaths and the US was still only halfway to its goal. And none of these vaccine-linked injuries, permanent disabilities, or deaths would have happened if we had followed the pandemic planning guidelines. So, these are all injuries and deaths *on top of the unnecessary deaths caused by "flattening the curve"*. These injuries and deaths are not inconsequential. These are real people, not numbers on a screen.

Vaccination is never a guaranteed zero-risk medical procedure, regardless of its benefits. So, why are people who have already had COVID not being excluded from vaccination in order to shield them from exposure to this demonstrable risk? By the end of May, over 20% of US blood donors (Health Day News, March 17, 2021) already had antibodies to the SARS-CoV-2 virus. Why aren't antibody tests being used to exclude people with antibodies from the vaccination rollout? And what about those who have cross-reactive immunity from previous exposure to one of the other coronaviruses (Majdoubi et al., 2021) that have been circulating in our communities long before COVID arrived? Any death or permanent disability among these people is not collateral damage -

they were fooled into taking a completely unneeded risk. That is not "justifiable risk".

All of these people already have immunity, so they had no risk to offset by further exposing themselves to the potential risks of immunization. People with pre-existing immunity are not a small percentage of the population. Up to 80% of people in Germany already have this pre-existing cross-reactive immunity (Nelde et al., June 17, 2020), though it varies greatly from country to country (Swiss Policy Research, September 2020). In other words, vaccination (and its associated risks) could be reduced by up to 80% simply by doing antibody testing and testing for cross-reactive immunity. And that's on top of the millions who have already had COVID and recovered.

Back in October of 2020, before the 2nd wave, the WHO already estimated that over 750 million people world-wide had already been infected (CNBC Health and Science, October 5, 2020)! Encouraging anyone to expose themselves to a known risk, however small it may be, when that person has no risk whatsoever to offset, is a criminal offence under the principles laid out by the Nuremberg Code. This demonstrates yet again the sheer recklessness and lack of nuance in the government's actions during this crisis. The goal is not to "get as many jabs into as many arms as possible". No matter how we look at this, every injury or death from this vaccine in a person who has already had COVID, or has antibodies, or has pre-existing immunity is unacceptable.

This should serve as a warning to those who administer the vaccine. If someone with pre-existing immunity is injured or dies from this vaccine, they can be held personally and criminally liable for that injury or death, as outlined by the Nuremberg Code[7], because we knew beforehand that this category of people exists, that it is possible to identify and sort them from the rest of the population, and that the vaccine offers no benefits that they didn't already have. They had no risk to offset. For them, the only thing the vaccine accomplished was to expose them to a new and entirely unnecessary risk, however small, of a vaccine-caused injury of death.

Anyone being offered this vaccine without being fully informed of its emergency use authorization (EUA), the unknown risks that go along with an EUA designation, the lack of long-term studies, a personalized risk/benefit calculation, the pointlessness of it if you already have immunity, and the small number of injuries and deaths documented on VAERS is a victim of coercion. Informed consent requires all of this knowledge, along with the context to understand it. Anything less is a violation of the Nuremberg Code.

And why is the government even offering the vaccine to children when they have the statistical equivalent of zero risk from this virus? As we learned from Dr. Henry's propaganda story, as of April 19th, 2021, only a single individual under the age of 30 had died with or from COVID in British Columbia. And that infant had pre-existing conditions. So, *a single vaccine-linked death in British Columbia of a healthy individual without pre-existing conditions under the age of 30 would make the vaccine more lethal than the virus to those under 30s in British Columbia.* Are these facts being shared as part of "informed consent"?

Every vaccine, like all medical interventions, should be evaluated on a case-by-case basis. Every person will have a different calculus depending on their age, on their pre-existing conditions, and on the risk posed by where they live and the nuanced details of how they live their lives. One-size-fits-all risk assessment is silly.

Yet the government has not disclosed how many people have pre-existing health conditions in each of the COVID death age categories. Vaccination of the healthy only makes sense if the healthy are being bowled over in large numbers by this virus. Everything in this investigative report shows that is not the case.

The outbreak data discussed earlier provided a much-needed glimpse into how badly our sense of personal risk from this virus has been distorted and how tone-deaf the government policies are. Context matters and there is an awful lot of missing context to the story provided by the government without which informed consent is simply not possible *for anyone*. Misrepresenting risk is a violation of the Nuremberg Code.

In a free society, it's not up to someone else to decide what risks you should be forced to take. And it is not acceptable to coerce anyone into a personal medical decision. We are not cattle to be shepherded into compliance. Yet health officials have worked very hard to ensure that the complete picture has been absent and now they expect us to accept vaccination based on the incomplete and distorted perception of risk they have created. That does not lead to informed consent.

In a rational world, until there was a vaccine available that could offer individual protection to the vulnerable, the goal should have been to create a ring of immune individuals around the pockets of vulnerable living among us. Population-wide lockdowns prevented that from happening. But once individual immunity became available through the pointy end of a syringe, the need to create a ring of herd immunity around the vulnerable dissolved because the vaccine gave everyone, including the vulnerable, the *option* to acquire individual protection, completely irrespective of what their neighbors do.

18 — Bypassing Parental Guardianship: Do Children Really Understand Their Risks Without Parental Oversight?

The obsession with this vaccine as the way to end the crisis has reached the point where the government is pushing to vaccinate children as young as 12 and allowing them to do so *without parental consent*. This opens the door to educators and health officials being able to pressure kids at school into taking it without their parents' consent (figure 46 and 47) and even without their parents' knowledge (figure 48):

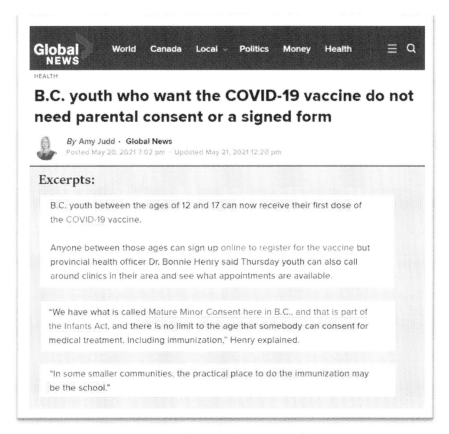

Figure 46: Vaccination of children aged 12 to 17 does not require parental consent for vaccination with an emergency-authorized vaccine (Global News, May 20, 2021)

And so it goes all around the country:

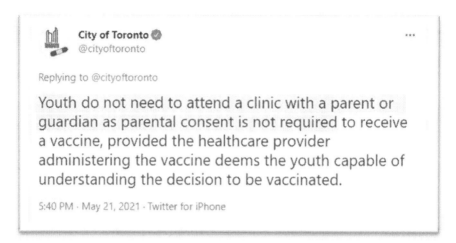

Figure 47: City of Toronto (Twitter, May 21, 2021)

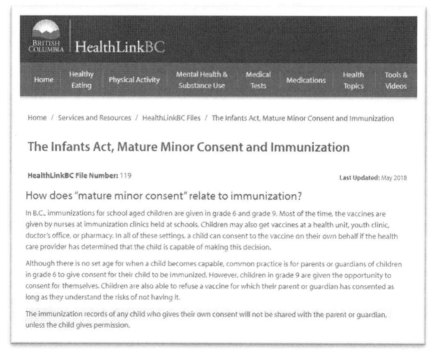

Figure 48: Parents will not be informed of a child's vaccination without the child's consent. Infants Act, Mature Minor Consent and Immunization, HealthLink BC (BC CDC, May 2018)

Are 12-year-olds mature enough to make those kinds of decisions without any parental input? Considering how one-sided the government's information campaign has been and how it has systematically avoided engaging in meaningful two-way public debate with critics, I even question whether most adults know the right questions to ask to be able to adequately inform themselves of their personal risks and benefits if they take this vaccine. If you were surprised by anything you read in this investigative report (I certainly ran across quite a few surprises while researching it), then you did not have all the information needed to give informed consent. Yet we are supposed to pretend that children have enough background knowledge to tease out all these nuanced details and know what questions to ask when figures of authority - teachers and health officials - are pushing them to make the "right" choice?

A child reaching a conclusion desired by an adult in a position of authority is not evidence that this child followed the same independent thought processes that an adult would follow in order to reach those conclusions, especially when the potential for coercive pressure exists. Children are not fully mature little adults with mature brains and a long history of life experiences to draw upon. They are easily influenced, impulsive, impatient, and often blind to the long-term ramifications of their actions. It's part of growing up.

Parental guardianship is meant give them an advocate to fill in the gaps, both to protect them and to help them acquire the perspective and maturity they will need in order to navigate the adult world. Society recognizes this fundamental concept of *growing into maturity* through our alcohol and drug consumption laws, sexual consent laws, voting age, military service age, and even in criminal law when prosecuting under-age offenders. Yet we are being asked to participate in a collective mass delusion by pretending that vaccination, with potentially life-changing or life-ending consequences (as shown by the VAERS data) is somehow different when it comes to children being able to understand the far-reaching ramifications of their decisions.

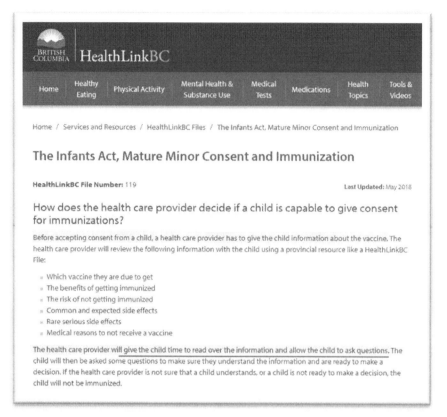

Figure 49: Parents will not be informed of a child's vaccination without the child's consent. Infants Act, Mature Minor Consent and Immunization, HealthLink BC (BC CDC, May 2018)

And we're supposed to also buy into the collective fantasy that government will not use coercion to pursue an agenda and that the power imbalance between children and teachers/health officials will not influence their decisions. It does not require an intention to coerce on the part of the adults - the goal may be perfectly well-meaning. But the power imbalance should, at a minimum, require the child to have another adult advocate on their side to counterbalance that one-sided relationship. The parent would seem like the most ideally suited, least likely to have their own agenda, and most likely to know the individual circumstances of the child's medical risks and have their best interests at heart.

Does this information campaign distributed to children in Saskatchewan look like coercion to you?

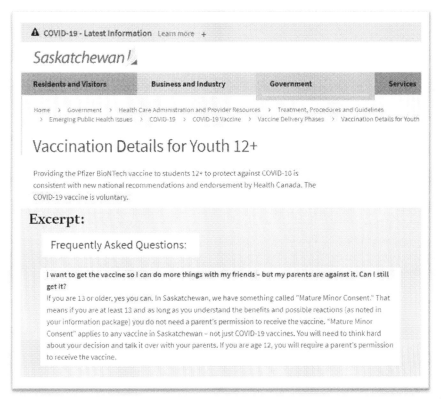

Figure 50: Vaccination details for youths 12+ being distributed by the Government of Saskatchewan (Government of Saskatchewan, May 20, 2021). Is this coercion?

It's rather ironic really; the recent #MeToo movement went as far as compelling society to question whether consent can be given freely in sexual encounters *between adults* when one of those adults is in a position of authority over the other (Schneebaum, Spring 2015). Yet we're supposed to pretend that there is no risk of coercion or abuse of authority (intentional or otherwise) when teachers and health officials are encouraging children as young as 12 to get vaccinated, particularly in a school environment where these figures of authority are able to have these conversations with children away from the oversight of their parents and where peer pressure from their friends is highly likely to influence their decisions.

Parental guardianship is a foundational legal concept in a free society to protect children from themselves and to protect children from other people with an agenda. The parent is the most likely member of society that will act in a child's best interests. Not all parents are perfect, but the alternative of allowing the government to erase this concept of parental guardianship and assume that role for children is far more dangerous. If ever there was a slippery slope, this is it. It doesn't take rocket science to understand all the other areas in which parental consent might interfere with a government's agenda or where a government bureaucrat might invest less time than parents would to study what's right for each individual child. Parental guardianship is a principle, not an outcome. What is being done under the umbrella of COVID hysteria is setting an extremely dangerous legal precedent. And it is being pushed on society without public consultation, without public debate, and without parliamentary transparency. The repercussions of this re-imaging of boundaries within society will be with us long after the virus fades out of sight.

Section 1 of the Nuremberg Code[8] explicitly states that: *"The voluntary consent of the human subject is absolutely essential. This means that the person involved should have the legal capacity to give consent; should be so situated as to be able to exercise free power of choice, without the intervention off any element of force, fraud, deceit, duress, overreaching, or other ulterior form of constraint or coercion; and should have sufficient knowledge and comprehension of the elements of the subject matter involved as to enable him to make an understanding and enlightened decision."*

Teachers and health care workers administering these vaccinations should pay attention. The Nuremberg Code also explicitly states: *"The duty and responsibility for ascertaining the quality of the consent rests upon each individual who initiates, directs, or engages in the experiment. It is a personal duty and responsibility which may not be delegated to another with impunity."*

As long as these vaccines remain under emergency use authorization and as long as we wait for long-term safety trials to be completed, these vaccines are, by definition, an experimental vaccine. The people administering these vaccines and those engaging in coercion, intentionally or not, can each be held *personally* accountable for human rights violations for their roles in this experiment. The take-home lesson from the Nuremberg Trials in the aftermath of World War II was that accountability for human rights violations does not stop with those giving the orders; accountability also extends to those carrying them out.

19 — When Government Goes "All-In" on One Strategy, All Others Are Pushed Aside: The Sorry Tale of Ivermectin and Its Unpopular Friends.

The moment the government committed to the vaccine another deadly snowball was set in motion. An emergency use authorization is not allowed if there are other treatment options available. Here is the US Food & Drug Administration explaining the issue:

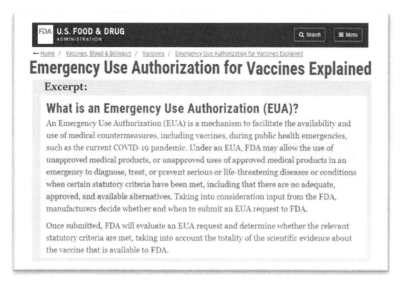

Figure 51: The US FDA's rules for emergency use authorization (US Food and Drug Administration, November 20, 2020). Canada's rules are a little different, but the underlying principle is the same.

There are hundreds of promising studies published on Ivermectin, bromhexine, hydroxychloroquine, vitamin D, and countless others, both for treatment and to use as a prophylaxis to prevent COVID. Off-label repurposing of drugs is a common practice, and safety testing is far easier and faster than developing new treatments. You only need to demonstrate effectiveness because their long-term side effects are already known. Yet government delays, arbitrary rules, and other restrictions are blocking these alternatives or hamstringing them with red tape at every turn. If they do work (and many show *a lot* of promise), the vaccine would lose its emergency use authorization.

But here's the multi-billion-dollar question: what if there was no known alternative when the emergency use authorization was proposed as a way to speed up vaccine development, but alternatives emerged shortly afterwards when the vaccine was already in development? Would the emergency use authorization be withdrawn? How would you compensate the vaccine makers, which have locked our governments into binding contracts, if they have to abandon ship mid-way into development or distribution? We'll never find out because all these alternatives are being systematically stonewalled by our government. Perhaps the paperwork will come through the day after the last vaccine is divvied out. Or perhaps not, since they're already talking about annual booster shots, ad infinitum.

It would be an embarrassment of incalculable proportions if a 40-year-old repurposed out-of-patent drug like Ivermectin, on the WHO's list of essential medicines and costing only a few dollars per dose, were to turn out to be as effective as the vaccine (Ivmmeta.com, May 18, 2021). So, in the interests of informed consent, here is a screengrab of a meta-analysis of 56 studies evaluating Ivermectin for COVID use - early treatment, late treatment, and for preventative (prophylaxis) treatment. Food for thought. If it is as effective as the numbers promise, every vaccination is illegal and every death caused by them is a crime, regardless of whether they signed the consent form or not.

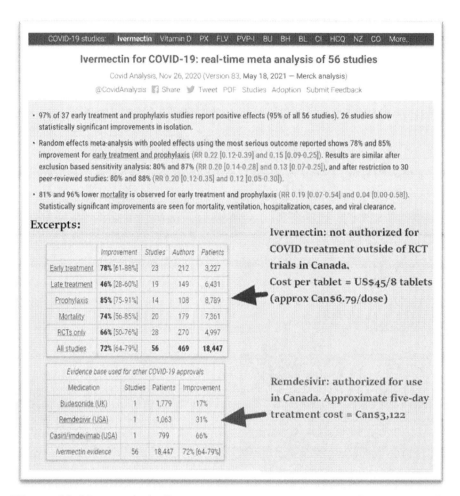

Figure 52: Meta analysis (Ivmmeta.com, May 18, 2021) of Ivermectin for COVID 19. Additional sources: Remdesivir policy in Canada (Government of Canada, January 29, 2021); Remdesivir cost per treatment (CATIE News, August 6, 2020); Ivermectin policy on the BC CDC website (BC Center for Disease Control, April 9, 2021); Cost of Ivermectin per dose (PharmacyChecker.com, January 12, 2021).

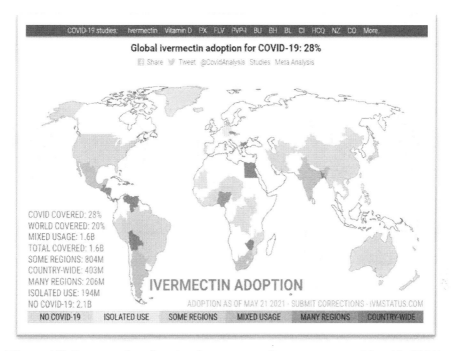

Figure 53: Ivermectin adoption by country (Ivmmeta.com, May 18, 2021).

This bizarre denial of any other possible ways of reducing risk to COVID even extends to Vitamin D. One of our Members of Parliament recently raised a question about the 75 peer-reviewed scientific studies showing the strong correlation between low vitamin D levels and severe outcomes from COVID. Our Minister of Health refused to address the essence of his question and instead simply condemned all these studies (7UMMIT Magazine, April 23, 2021) as "fake news". Yet it is a long-established fact (Zhou et al., August, 2018) that topping up Vitamin D levels reduces severe outcomes if you catch the flu. Britain went as far as supplementing its most vulnerable with Vitamin D (BBC News, November 28, 2020) during the pandemic. What did they have to lose?

How many more of our most vulnerable, prevented from going out into the sun during their forced isolation in nursing homes during COVID, could have been saved if everyone had been encouraged to take vitamin D supplements throughout the last two winters. It would have cost pennies per dose and there are unlikely to be side effects from a Vitamin D top-up (certainly none as severe as the vaccine!). But with everything riding on the vaccines (and lockdowns), most especially the reputations of the politicians and health officials who began promoting them, there really isn't room for anything else. Politics and special interests appear to be taking priority over "doing everything we can to keep you safe."

20 — The Lies…. Summary

The deliberate fear being spread by our health officials, politicians, and media is a vicious and irresponsible misrepresentation of risk. Not all outbreaks are created equal. Not all cases pose equal risk. The underlying vulnerability of individuals matters. Context matters.

Most vulnerable people are found in very specific settings: long-term care & hospitals. *Society-wide lockdowns don't work because the overwhelming majority of people at risk from this virus are already segregated from society.* Lockdowns don't add anything the vulnerable don't already have.

On the contrary, in addition to the deadly collateral damage caused by lockdowns, lockdowns also hold the vulnerable hostage to low rates of herd immunity in their communities, leaving them trapped in indefinite isolation and at risk of everyone they encounter. Many of the most vulnerable don't have 15 months to wait. Most long-term care residents have less than 5 months to live once they move into these government institutions. Instead of battening down the hatches for a single 6-to-8-week wave, these vulnerable are now forced to die in isolation, without the support of their loved ones to help them through the last difficult months of their lives. It is a cruel, terrifying, and undignified end. And it was entirely preventable if our government had just followed the protocols laid out in the pandemic planning guidelines and respected the constitutional rights and freedoms of its citizens. Pinning our hopes on a vaccine only stretched this nightmare out even longer, with deadly consequences. This adventure in DIY pandemic management needs to stop.

The vulnerable need focused protection and strong doors until this madness ends. The false promises of masks and social distancing are merely illusions of safety; policies that rely on them to protect the vulnerable are worse than doing nothing at all.

The rest of us need to set aside our fears, look at the government's own official numbers, stop listening to these propaganda artists, and remind ourselves that life is never risk-free. There are many other risks far worse than COVID, starting with the risk of being afraid to live our lives. It is time to start living again in a free and open society. The sooner we do, the sooner the vulnerable can do the same.

And what about the vaccines? We never should have held society hostage while we waited for them to arrive. But should they at least still be offered as a voluntary coercion-free option to those who want them?

The problem is this: the abhorrent absence of context, incomplete data, and intentionally distorted sense of risk cultivated by public health officials and by many in the scientific community, along with the systematic vilification of critics who tried to raise serious and credible concerns, as well as the absence of long-term safety trials to rule out the critics' worst fears, all these factors come together to raise doubts about whether anyone, including the most vulnerable, is able to fully understand and quantify their individual risk from COVID and objectively weigh that risk against the benefits and risks of vaccination. Informed consent is not possible against this backdrop.

And sadly, it is also questionable whether science in its current sorry state is even *capable* of answering the most basic questions about the safety of the vaccine. Everything we have witnessed over the past year and a half signals that our scientific institutions and many of those inside them have abandoned all the core principles that make science work. Their behavior has had far more in common with the slander, smears, shaming, and cancel culture tactics of an out-of-control kindergarten than with the distinguished forebearers of their professions upon whose shoulders they stand. These institutions are rotten to the core.

Are the vaccines safe? The mechanism that can lead us to an objective, nuanced, and robust answer to that question is broken. We must not allow ourselves to fall for the *sunk cost fallacy* and plow ever further into the unknown when we do not yet know the long-term consequences of the uncharted territories into which we are throwing ourselves. Which leaves us right back where we started. The pandemic planning guidelines. Because it's never too late to do the right thing.

~

I hope this guided tour through the pandemic and through the endless string of deadly scandals that the government has created has given you a sense of perspective and cleared a path through the fog of the past 18 months. The task now falls on each of us to help our fellow citizens climb down from their fear.

We need their voices to join ours, not only to regain our lives, but also to rekindle the appetite for a functioning democracy rooted in accountability, transparency, honest debate, and respect for individual rights. We also need to send a clear message to our leaders that the technical expertise of those working in scientific fields should never be confused with the broader process of scientific inquiry. As the experience of the past 18 months has shown, science ceases to function as a tool for revealing objective truth when society allows people in lab coats to use credentials and the illusion of consensus to silence their critics and to avoid transparency, evidence, context, and the gauntlet of debate.

So, please share this investigative report with friends, family members, neighbors, and co-workers to help them gain perspective over the nightmare we have all been living for the past 18 months. This ends only when the government loses the support of the crowd. This only ends when your neighbors are no longer afraid to come over for a BBQ, when your friends and family members are no longer afraid to give you a hug, and when the doctors, lawyers, and policemen, who are also members of our communities, recognize the gravity of the scandal that they have been drawn into. And so, in that vein, please also send this to every lawyer, policeman, elected representative, city councillor, judge, and journalist that you know. This nightmare world of fabricated lies only ends when communities stand up together and say, "Enough!"

~

I have made harsh calls for accountability throughout this long text. Human rights violations on this scale and with such a vast global death toll cannot be shrugged off. "We didn't know" is only true for the members of the public caught up in the panic. The science, the protocols, and our rights were never in doubt and, as I have demonstrated, those in charge were well aware of them from day 1. Do not let the magicians use the fog they created to escape into the night. We owe it to their victims, and we owe it to future generations to make sure that the evil that happened on our watch is rooted out so it can never happen again. Just because the media has ignored it does not reduce the enormity of the profound suffering and unnecessary dying that our leaders have caused.

The familiar faces that have held us hostage for the past 18 months may not look like monsters in jackboots, but it is important to remember that behind all the sterile numbers are real people. Those numbers represent children, grandparents, fathers, and mothers whose lives were cut short by these monsters' blatant lies, willful manipulation, reckless disregard for protocols, utter disrespect for human rights, and flagrant contempt for the principles of science and democracy, to which they are *sworn* in their professional roles. The numbers represent real people who leave behind real grieving loved ones. No emergency benefit cheque can replace them. Nothing can bring them back.

Despite the air of caring radiating from Dr. Henry's seemingly empathetic concern for our wellbeing, she was nonetheless willing to *knowingly* reduce the infant in her story to a mere propaganda tool. She hijacked the tragedy of its death to tell a lie that was the complete opposite of the lessons that should have been given to the public based on the actual facts surrounding its death.

And she is just one of thousands of health officials, scientists, and politicians across this country and around the world who have knowingly played this despicable game of deception. It is one thing to be swept up in mass hysteria. It is quite another to knowingly play chess with the truth and gamble with other people's lives in order to intentionally fuel hysteria to engineer some alleged "greater good". It is the height of hubris to be so certain of the righteousness of their cause that even the truth was merely an obstacle in their path.

These are not the actions of people with real empathy for their fellow citizens and an honest commitment to objective truth. Their patronizing lies of "good intentions" reveal the extent to which they view us as cattle to be herded into compliance and not as fellow equals in a free and open society. Those who abandon the principles of transparency, evidence, honest debate, and respect for the individual autonomy of their fellow citizens have abandoned the core principles that make science and democracy work. Without them, all that remains is tyranny over the bodies and minds of their subjects, all legitimized by an Orwellian Ministry of Truth. No-one has the right to manage their individual risk by controlling the lives of others. Those who are so certain that they know best that they are willing to strong-arm others into compliance are a threat to the very essence of what it means to live in a free and open society.

Dr. Henry's government, along with every other government at every level of politics, participated in a ruthless global social engineering experiment that may well have cost the life of the infant in Dr. Henry's propaganda story, and most certainly cost the lives of thousands (if not millions) all around the world who paid the ultimate price for governmental hubris and medical adventurism.

Perhaps it shouldn't surprise us that those who have their fingerprints on this disaster are so eager to blame the actions of ordinary citizens trying desperately to live their lives. The lonely pastor, the restauranteur, the hairdresser, and now all those who have chosen not to get vaccinated are easy targets when the machinery of government grinds into action in the interests of self-preservation in order to give the public an alternate scapegoat for 18 months of government-engineered Hell. By now it must be painfully obvious to these self-righteous monsters, no matter how much they allowed themselves to get swept up in the virtuous delusions of their own propaganda, that they are inching towards accountability in front of a human rights tribunal. The world is waking up. They can no longer prevent it.

The most horrendous crimes are often well hidden in a fog of confusion, disguised from its victims behind a shroud of good intentions and noble ideals. Most monsters don't fit the mold of what we imagine monsters to be. Most are loved by the very people they hurt. Most are driven by good intentions, a heightened sense of superiority, and an incapacity for self-reflection. Most are gradually transformed into monsters when they experience the heady intoxication of being given responsibility and control over the lives of others. Most are fueled by the thirst of adoration from a receptive crowd. And most are so convinced of the righteous of their actions and the need to sacrifice for the good of the herd that there is no stack of bodies too tall to climb over to achieve their "virtuous" goals.

But monsters do not appear out of a vacuum. They are created by an absence of limits when a permissive society exempts them from transparency, debate, and checks and balances. Monsters inevitably emerge when liberal democracy and the scientific process of inquiry cease to impose limits on a chosen elite living among us. Science and democracy *are* those limits. They *are* the processes that keep our darkest illiberal impulses in check. The past 18 months gave us a window into what a pre-Enlightenment worldview looks like, with modern technology at its fingertips and without the checks and balances imposed by scientific inquiry and liberal democracy. So, it is time to hold these monsters to account, not only in pursuit of justice for those they have hurt, but also to pull back the curtain to show society the illiberal world that it has been sleepwalking into.

I'm going to end the investigative report portion of this book with the face of Nancy Russell. She chose to end her life through assisted suicide rather than endure the forced isolation of a second lockdown. Never forget.

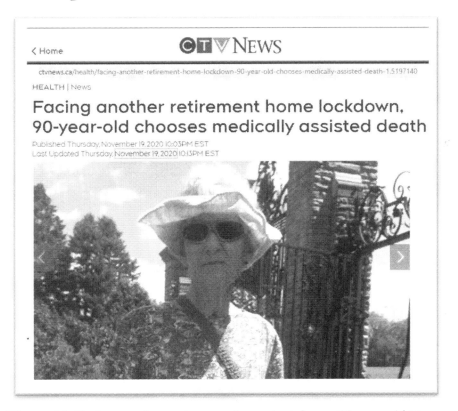

Figure 54: Facing another retirement home lockdown, 90-year-old Nancy Russell choses medically assisted death (CTV News, November 19th, 2020).

PART II —
Washington's Inoculation Gamble: Calculating the Vegas Odds of Virus vs Vax Risks, and the Goal of Herd Immunity

"Are you getting the vaccine?" I have had to disappoint a lot of friends and family when I tell them that I'm going to sit this one out; that I don't like the odds so I'm choosing to be part of the control group in this grand experiment. Furrowed brows, a sharp look of disapproval, and inevitably I hear some version of *"It's not about you, it's about saving lives by building a ring of immunity around the vulnerable to reduce the chance that they get infected."*

The problem with that argument is that it is fundamentally untrue. Vaccination is all about you. You're the one that has to decide if you want to offset the risk of the virus by taking a risk on vaccination. And you're the one that has to live with the consequences of that decision, whichever way you choose. It's a very personal decision that no-one can make for you.

Informed consent begins with a very basic risk calculation but, like almost everything else during this crisis, the government has gone to great lengths to avoid giving the public the relevant information to make an informed personal decision. So, I did what the government has refused to do: use the government's own official numbers to calculate your Vegas odds of death from the virus so you can weigh those odds against the risks of getting the jab. And I will show you how the concept of herd immunity is being willfully distorted to shame you into getting the jab, despite the fact that the vulnerable in this pandemic are all capable of getting their own.

21 — George Washington's Gamble

History provides fantastic examples to make concepts jump up out of a page, thus making a story easier to tell. So, I'm going to take you back to a time when vaccination was first being developed as a public health strategy in order to highlight all the key elements that are required for someone to make an informed risk-benefit calculation (your Vegas odds) and to show you how far our public health agencies have strayed from all the ethics and principles of vaccination.

In the early days of the Revolutionary War the smallpox virus followed American troops everywhere. Plague and pestilence always follow closely on the heels of war. Not only did smallpox spread like wildfire among George Washington's troops and tie up valuable resources to care for sick soldiers, it also caused his troops to spread smallpox to all the towns and villages along their path.

For children under 1 year of age, smallpox had a fatality rate of between 40 and 50%! For the population at large, the fatality rate was round 30%. Losing 30% of your troops even before you fight a single battle is unacceptable. And there is no way you can win a war if you turn the population against you by allowing the Grim Reaper to march into town alongside you because he will amuse himself by emptying the cradles of all the villages that you rely on to feed your troops. It's hard to win hearts and minds when those you claim to be fighting for are asked to bear the highest cost.

Smallpox came in two varieties - variola major (the common variety with the 30% death rate) and variola minor (with a death rate of around 1%). Surviving one gave immunity to the other. They were, in fact, the same virus. The difference was how the virus began its assault on the body. If it entered the body through the air (via the respiratory system), it would spread through the body via the lymphatic system, which led to the lethal variola major version of the disease. But if it entered the body via a scratch on the skin, it led to a more local and less lethal variola minor infection, which allowed the patient to develop immunity without the virus spreading through the lymphatic system.

Early smallpox inoculation utilized a strategy called variolation to purposely infect people with variola minor by introducing pus from an infected individual into scratches on their skin. Acquiring immunity using variolation still caused a death rate of 1%. That's almost 10x more deadly than our current COVID virus (Swiss Policy Research, September 2020), even before accounting for the difference in COVID risk caused by age and pre-existing health conditions. Variolation was a dangerous and hellish experience, yet many people considered it a justifiable risk because smallpox was so deadly and so common.

No-one was asked to take that risk for someone else. Variolation, like all immunization, was about individuals weighing their personal risks of immunization against their personal risk from the disease.

John Adams, Founding Father and 2nd US President, described his own experience with variolation:

"Do not conclude from any Thing I have written that I think Inoculation a light matter -- A long and total abstinence from everything in Nature that has any Taste; two long heavy Vomits, one heavy Cathartic, four and twenty Mercurial and Antimonial Pills, and, three weeks of Close Confinement to an House, are, according to my Estimation, no small matters."

Eventually variolation was replaced by a much less risky alternative when the world's first vaccine was developed using the closely related and much less dangerous cowpox virus to induce immunity against smallpox. The word *vaccination* comes from the Latin word *Vacca,* which means cow. But at the time that George Washington was fighting the Revolutionary War, variolation was the only option.

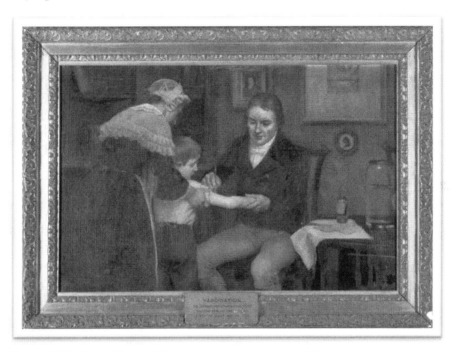

Figure 55: Dr. Edward Jenner created the world's first vaccine - the smallpox vaccine - because he knew that dairy workers who contracted cowpox (a relatively mild infection) were immune to smallpox. This painting captures his first experimental vaccination on a boy by the name of James Phipps on May 14th, 1796.

George Washington was initially extremely reluctant to inoculate his troops because of how dangerous variolation was, but he eventually recognized that *"we should have more to dread from it [smallpox], than from the Sword of the Enemy."* One study suggests that for every American soldier killed by the British, the Americans were losing ten of their own soldiers to some sort of disease (Brenda Thacker, The Washington Library). And so, George Washington quarantined his troops (to prevent the variolation process from sparking an epidemic in the surrounding community) and inoculated them (under a cover of absolute secrecy to prevent the British from attacking while his quarantined troops were bedridden).

Variolation allowed George Washington to give his troops *individual* protection against the virus, thus giving him an advantage in war. And it allowed him to protect the villages that he depended on for food by drying up the source of viral spread. In other words, inoculating his troops for their own protection also allowed him to protect the vulnerable babies in their cradles. And the reason it was ethical to try to create herd immunity to protect babies in their cradles was because those taking the risk of variolation (his soldiers) were also getting a benefit for themselves that outweighed their risk from variolation.

Variolation leveled the playing field against the British, many of which were arriving on American soil with immunity because of prior inoculation or natural exposure (Brenda Thacker, The Washington Library) back in Britain. George Washington's gamble ultimately played a huge role in why the Stars and Stripes and not the Union Jack flies over American soil today.

22 — Calculating Your Vegas Odds

Vaccination is a lot like sports betting, except that you have three sets of odds to calculate. First there is the odds of death if you catch the virus. In George Washington's time, the odds of death if you were infected with smallpox were roughly 1 in 3. Catching smallpox was a game of Russian Roulette with a three-chambered gun and one live round of ammo.

The second calculation is the odds of losing your life (or becoming permanently disabled) during vaccination. No vaccine is 100% risk-free because *"each person's body reacts to vaccines differently"* (CDC, n.d.). Variolation was a game of Russian Roulette with 100 chambers and only one live round. Definitely better odds than full-blown smallpox, but not something to take lightly either.

Despite the light-hearted reference to Vegas odds, this isn't a casino where you can keep your bets small to ensure that you can keep playing if you lose on your first turn. A vaccination, like an infection with the actual disease, are both one-time bets. You're betting the farm. It's your life on the line. And there's no opting out of the game because, by refusing to bet on one, you automatically place your bets on the other.

The odds faced by George Washington's troops favored variolation. 1 in 100 vs 1 in 3. But everyone's personal exposure to the risk matters too - that's the third calculation everyone has to make before getting vaccinated. George Washington's troops were almost certain to get exposed at some point because of the cramped unhygienic conditions of war and their constant mingling with strangers. It only takes one soldier to bring the virus back to the barracks after a wild night out on the town and the whole division gets put at risk. A rural hermit has a very different calculation, not because he's not at risk if he gets exposed, but because he has a much lower chance of getting exposed in the first place. Calculating your odds is a very individual process.

The risk posed by COVID, like most respiratory viruses, is not evenly distributed across society. Lifestyle plays a big role in your risk of exposure. Long-term care residents and staff working in hospitals or nursing homes face orders of magnitude more risk of exposure than a retired person living at home, someone working from home, a truck driver, or farmer out in his fields. Some people are certain to be exposed to the virus at some point, possibly even to high viral loads. Others may go a lifetime without ever crossing paths with it.

While everyone has to gauge these highly individual factors for themselves, it's nevertheless possible to put some numbers on how age and underlying conditions affect your risk from the virus and to compare those numbers to the risk of death or serious injury from the vaccines. It's time to calculate some Vegas odds for the virus and for the vax.

23 — The Calculations: Vegas Odds of Death from COVID

<u>Step 1 - Infection Fatality Rate</u>: In the following chart I've calculated the odds of death from a COVID infection using the CDC's official infection fatality rate for each age category (this is the risk of death IF someone catches an infection). Clearly age matters a lot. But before these odds can give you any meaningful insights about your personal level of risk, we need to refine those numbers to account for:

- the portion of the population that has pre-existing cross-reactive immunity and is therefore not at risk of catching the disease in the first place,

- the level of community exposure required to reach herd immunity,

- and pre-existing health conditions.

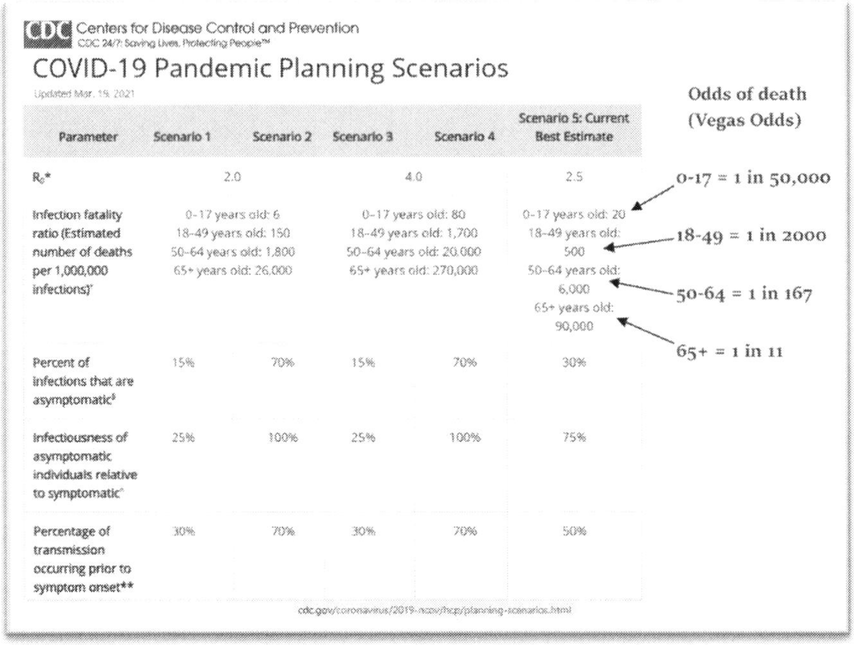

Parameter	Scenario 1	Scenario 2	Scenario 3	Scenario 4	Scenario 5: Current Best Estimate
R_0*	2.0		4.0		2.5
Infection fatality ratio (Estimated number of deaths per 1,000,000 infections)†	0-17 years old: 6 18-49 years old: 150 50-64 years old: 1,800 65+ years old: 26,000		0-17 years old: 80 18-49 years old: 1,700 50-64 years old: 20,000 65+ years old: 270,000		0-17 years old: 20 18-49 years old: 500 50-64 years old: 6,000 65+ years old: 90,000
Percent of infections that are asymptomatic§	15%	70%	15%	70%	30%
Infectiousness of asymptomatic individuals relative to symptomatic^	25%	100%	25%	100%	75%
Percentage of transmission occurring prior to symptom onset**	30%	70%	30%	70%	50%

Figure 56: Calculating the odds of death from a COVID infection based on the CDC's official numbers (US CDC, March 19, 2021) (to check my math here is an example for the 0-17 group: 1,000,000÷20 = 50,000=1:50,000)

<u>Step 2 -Accounting for cross-reactive antibodies (T-cell immunity)</u>: Research studies have demonstrated that many people have cross-reactive T-cell immunity to COVID-19 because of prior exposure to other coronaviruses. A previous encounter with one of COVID's closely related cousins is a serious advantage. It varies from country to country; however, a range of studies from around the world shows that from 6% to 81% of adults and up to 60% of children (Swiss Policy Research, September 2021) already have this cross-reactive immunity. A study from British Columbia published by the US National Center for Biotechnical Information found that 90% to 99% of adults in the Vancouver area show positive antibody reactivity for the SARS-CoV-2 spike, RBD, or the N antigen (Majdoubi et al., 2021). And an article published in the British Medical Journal (Doshi, 2020) referenced 6 studies

demonstrating T-cell reactivity against SARS-CoV-2 in 20% to 50% of people with no known exposure to the virus. This last article makes several important points about cross-reactive T cell immunity:

- *"SARS-CoV-1 reactive T cells were found in SARS patients 17 years after infection."* Thus, the public health messaging that we need booster shots every year against COVID-19 flies in the face of evidence from SARS-CoV-2's closely related coronavirus cousin. Antibodies from an infection may fade relatively quickly but we can expect T-cell immunity from a prior infection to continue to provide protection for a long time.

- The study also points out lessons learned during the 2009 H1N1 pandemic. Data on B-cells and, in particular, T-cells, which are *"known to blunt disease severity"*, forced a change in views at the WHO and CDC *"from an assumption before 2009 that most people will have no immunity to the pandemic virus' to one that acknowledged that **the vulnerability of a population to a pandemic virus is related in part to the level of pre-existing immunity to the virus.**"* [my emphasis]

Cross-reactive immunity is not an on-off switch but would be best thought of as a scale. Some people will be sufficiently protected by this cross-reactive immunity to be entirely protected from symptomatic disease, others will nonetheless become ill or even be hospitalized, particularly if they have a weak immune system as a result of pre-existing health conditions. But these cross-reactive antibodies would go a long way towards explaining why SARS-CoV-2 leads to asymptomatic infections in the vast majority of people, severe outcomes in people who have weak immunity, and only affects a small number of people without pre-existing conditions, presumably those who do not have this cross-reactive immunity.

The presence of cross-reactive antibodies has two implications. It implies that we are far closer to herd immunity than if this virus was entirely unrelated to other coronaviruses already circulating in the community. And it demands that we reassess the odds of death or serious injury from SARS-CoV-2 in order to reflect this pre-existing immunity. So, even if we assume an entirely theoretical middle-of-the-road estimate of 20% of people having no risk of disease because of pre-existing cross-reactive immunity, the odds would change as follows:

COVID odds of death (Vegas Odds) by age, adjusted for cross-reactive immunity for 20% of the population.

0-17 = 1 in 62,500

18-49 = 1 in 2500

50-64 = 1 in 208

65+ = 1 in 14

Figure 57: COVID odds of death by age, adjusted for cross-reactive immunity. (To check my math here is an example for the 0-17 group: 1,000,000 ÷ (100%-20%) ÷ 20 = 62,500 = 1:62,500)

Step 3 - Accounting for your chance of being infected before we reach herd immunity: Once a community reaches herd immunity, the virus is essentially starved of available hosts and cannot keep spreading. Again, let's use a conservative estimate that says herd immunity will be reached when 90% of the population achieves some kind of immunity, either through infection, vaccination, or cross-reactive immunity. If you don't catch the virus before that 90% herd immunity level is reached, you probably won't catch it because the virus won't be spreading anymore. Let's adjust the numbers again:

COVID odds of death (Vegas Odds) by age, adjusted for cross-reactive immunity for 20% of the population AND herd immunity being reached at 90%

0-17 = 1 in 69,444

18-49 = 1 in 2777

50-64 = 1 in 231

65+ = 1 in 15

Figure 58: COVID odds of death by age, adjusted for cross-reactive immunity and a herd immunity target of 90%. (To check my math here is an example for the 0-17 group: 1,000,000 ÷ (100%-20%) ÷ 90% ÷ 20 = 69,444=1:69,444)

Step 4 - Accounting for pre-existing conditions: Those with a severe pre-existing health condition face a much higher risk than those who don't. The US CDC is happy to tell you all the pre-existing health conditions that accompany COVID deaths, but a clear breakdown by age has been extraordinarily difficult to find. However, an obscure report released by Statistics Canada last winter did just that and, since the virus doesn't care what passport you carry, Canada's numbers are good enough for the brute calculations I'm doing to guestimate our Vegas odds:

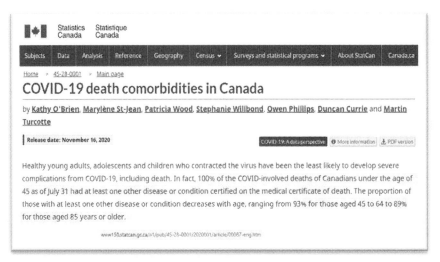

Figure 59: COVID-19 death comorbidities in Canada (Statistics Canada, November 16, 2020). *"100% of the COVID-involved deaths of Canadians under the age of 45 as of July 31 had at least one other disease or condition certified on the medical certificate of death."*

Remarkably, 100% of all Canadian deaths under the age of 45 had comorbidities - they were already sick with something else *before catching COVID!* (I know the US age brackets don't overlap exactly with the Canadian data, but it's close enough; Vegas odds aren't precision engineering, they are ballpark rules of thumb). So... if you are healthy and under the age of 45, you have ZERO statistical risk of death if you catch COVID. If you fall in this category, vaccination might at most spare you a nasty flu-like ordeal, but vaccination will not reduce your risk of death since that risk is already at zero.

Let that sink in! *Hundreds of millions* of people around the world are being encouraged to risk their life on these vaccines without having any risk of COVID death to offset. For these people, the vaccine is, quite literally, more dangerous than the virus. They get to play a version of Russian Roulette where they still face the risk of finding that live round of ammo when they spin the cylinder and pull the trigger, but there is no prize to be won if they survive the challenge.

Anyone under the age of 45 who does not have pre-existing health conditions is being asked to take this vaccine purely to reduce someone else's risk from this virus - for herd immunity - despite the fact that all those who are vulnerable are now able to protect themselves with the jab (more on that later). It's like being asked to undergo variolation, with all its risks, without being at risk from smallpox. Imagine George Washington forcing that on his troops - they all would have mutinied or deserted.

Let's adjust the Vegas Odds again using the US statistics for the percentage of people living with multiple chronic health conditions (shown in the chart below) and the Canadian comorbidity statistics:

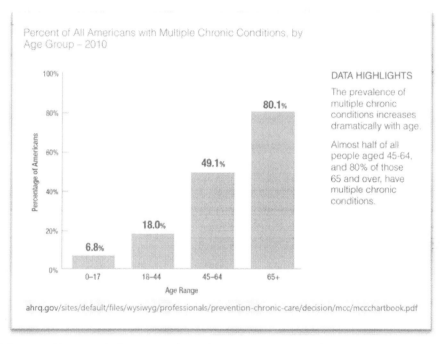

Figure 60: People living with multiple chronic conditions by age group (Agency for Healthcare Research and Quality, April 2014)

Here is the giant data table I used to calculate the Vegas odds, layer by layer. The take-home odds, by age group and health status, are shown in bold the bottom row:

Calculating the Vegas Odds of Death from COVID, by Age Group

Age Groups	0 - 17	18 - 49	50 - 64	+65
Deaths per Million (from CDC) DPM	20	500	6,000	90,000
Starting Population	1,000,000	1,000,000	1,000,000	1,000,000
Vegas Odds	50,000	2,000	167	11
Pop. adjustment for Cross-reactive Immunity (20%)	1,250,000	1,250,000	1,250,000	1,250,000
Vegas Odds	62,500	2,500	208	14
Pop. adjustment for Herd Immunity reached at 90%	1,388,889	1,388,889	1,388,889	1,388,889
Vegas Odds	69,444	2,778	231	15
Population living with multiple chronic conditions	6.8%	18.0%	49.1%	80.1%

Age Groups SPLIT	0-17 (without pre-existing health conditions)	0-17 (with pre-existing health conditions)	18-49 (without pre-existing health conditions)	18-49 (with pre-existing health conditions)	50-64 (without pre-existing health conditions)	50-64 (with pre-existing health conditions)	+65 (without pre-existing health conditions)	+65 (with pre-existing health conditions)
Population with pre-existing conditions	1,294,444	94,444	1,138,889	250,000	706,944	681,944	276,389	1,112,500
Deaths with Comorbidities DWC	0.0%	100.0%	0.0%	100.0%	7.0%	93.0%	11.0%	89.0%
Deaths per Million by underlying health (DPMxDWC)	0	20	0	500	420	5,580	9,900	80,100
➤ Vegas Odds	zero risk	1 : 4,722	zero risk	1 : 500	1 : 1,683	1 : 122	1 : 28	1 : 14

Figure 61: Calculating the Vegas Odds of Death from COVID, by age group, adjusted for cross-reactive immunity, a herd immunity target of 90%, and pre-existing health conditions. The bottom row shows the take-home odds by age category and health conditions.

And these odds could easily be refined still further by the type and severity of various pre-existing health conditions. For example, a June 1st study published in *The Lancet Diabetes and Endocrinology* called *"Associations between body-mass index and COVID-19 severity in 6.9 million people in England: a prospective, community-based, cohort study"* (Gao et al., 2021) demonstrated that risk of severe outcomes increased substantially as body fat exceeds the healthy range (or if body fat fell below the healthy weight range), so much so that one of the study's conclusions was that *"Our findings from this large population-based cohort emphasize that excess weight is associated with substantially increased risks of severe COVID-19 outcomes, and one of the most important modifiable risk factors identified to date."*

In other words, not only does your risk vary based on the kinds of pre-existing health conditions you have, but your risk increases further the further your body mass is from your ideal weight (in other words, your risk increases both if you are underweight and if you are overweight). But the good news is that it gives you a great deal of control over your level of risk from the virus by making sure that you get your body mass into a healthy range. Figure 62, taken from the study's supplementary appendix illustrates how risk varies with body mass index:

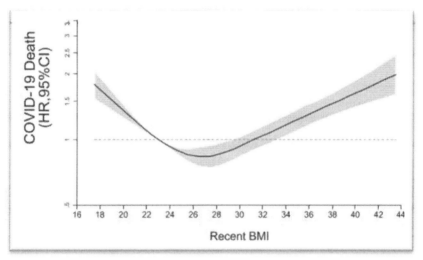

Figure 62: Associations of Body Mass Index (BMI) with COVID-19 deaths (Gao et al., 2021). In other words, the further you are from your ideal weight (either overweight or underweight), the greater your risk of death from COVID.

And figure 63, taken from the same study's supplementary appendix, shows how strong the correlation is between severe outcomes and body mass index for various age groups with various body mass indices. As an example of how to read the chart, 93% of the risk of death from COVID in people aged 20-39 with a body mass index of 40 can be explained by their body mass index. 93%! You can also see from the chart that this correlation between body fat levels and severe outcomes is strongest among the young and gets weaker in older age groups. In other words, for those who are young and obese, most of their risk from COVID is because of their obesity. For those who are old and obese, obesity increases their risk but their age nonetheless also plays a big role in their level of risk (immune systems get weaker with age).

COVID-19 Hospital admission	Incidence rate per 10,000 population	Attributable fractions % per 10,000 person-year			
		BMI 23 kg/m²	BMI 30 kg/m²	BMI 35 kg/m²	BMI 40 kg/m²
20-39 years	0.040	0	45	64	77
40-59 years	0.120	0	42	60	73
60-79 years	0.316	0	24	38	49
80+ years	1.141	0	7	11	16
COVID-19 ICU admission					
20-39 years	0.005	0	57	77	87
40-59 years	0.025	0	52	71	83
60-79 years	0.049	0	29	44	56
80+ years	0.025	0	33	50	63
COVID-19 Death					
20-39 years	0.001	0	67	85	93
40-59 years	0.016	0	57	77	87
60-79 years	0.121	0	19	30	39
80+ years	0.765	0	0	0	0

Figure 63: Attributable risks and fractions in risk of severe COVID-19 outcomes (hospitalization, ICU admission, and death) associated with body mass index (BMI) across age groups (Adapted from Gao et al., 2021).

With body fat levels playing such a big role in the level of risk to COVID, isn't it ironic that gyms were among the first businesses that were shuttered when this madness began even as the junk food aisle stayed open.

On their own, the Vegas odds of death from the virus are already rather shocking and give some perspective on just how irresponsible and unethical a mass vaccine rollout is for the millions who don't need it. It also highlights how different the risk is for different age groups and health categories. But for those who do face a risk from the virus, they also need to understand their Vegas odds of death or serious injury from the vaccines. Imagine George Washington's soldiers submitting to variolation without knowing if variolation or the virus posed the greater risk. The devil is always hidden in the details (and in the fine print).

24 — The Calculations: Vegas Odds of Death or Injury from the Vaccines

To calculate your Vegas odds of injury or death from the vaccines I used the data from the UK's vaccination program, which reports adverse drug reactions (ADRs) through their Yellow Card system (MHRA-GOV.UK, n.d.). These numbers were aggregated in a sobering report published on June 9th by the Evidence-based Medicine Consultancy Ltd (Lawrie, 2021), which gives us an insight into the severity of the adverse events being reported. As President John Adams would say, they are no small matter. Nor does surviving the game of Russian Roulette with the vaccine mean that your ordeal is over. I encourage you to read the full report because the range of injuries, many with life-long debilitating consequences, is staggering.

I have summarized some of the key numbers and quotes for you below to give you a sense of what you are risking when you take the vaccine. And then I will use these numbers to calculate the Vegas odds of a vaccine-linked injury or death.

UK COVID Vaccinations as of May 6th, 2021:

- 39 million single doses and 24 million both doses (for a total of 63,000,000 doses)
- 1253 deaths (total).
- 888,196 adverse drug reactions, including 256,224 individual reports.

Bleeding, Clotting, and Ischemic Reactions ("Ischemic" is a medical term that means some part of your body is not getting enough blood supply and is therefore being deprived of oxygen, like the heart, brain, or any other part of your body): 13,766 events (856 fatal)

- *"Our analysis indicates that thromboembolic ADRs have been reported in almost every vein and artery, including large vessels like the aorta, and in every organ including other parts of the brain, lungs, heart, spleen, kidneys, ovaries and liver, with life-threatening and life-changing consequences. The most common Yellow Card categories affected by these sorts of ADRs were the nervous system (152 fatalities, mainly from brain bleeds and clots), respiratory (with 103 fatalities, mainly from pulmonary thromboembolism) and cardiac categories (81 fatalities)."*

Immune System Adverse Drug Reactions (Infection, Inflammation, Autoimmune, Allergic): 54,870 events (171 fatal)

- *"Among 1,187 people for whom post-vaccination COVID infection was reported, there were 72 fatalities"*
- *"Many 'INFECTION' category ADRs indicated the occurrence of re-activation of latent viruses, including Herpes Zoster or shingles (1,827 ADRs), Herpes Simplex (943 ADRs, 1 fatal), and Rabies (1 fatal ADR) infections. This is strongly suggestive of vaccine-induced immune-compromise."*
- *"Also suggestive of vaccine-induced immunocompromise was the high number of immune-mediated reported, including Guillain-Barre Syndrome (280 ADRs, 6 deaths), Crohn's and non-infective colitis, (231 ADRs, 2 deaths) and Multiple Sclerosis (113 ADRs)"*
- *"Allergic responses to the vaccines comprised 25,270 reported ADRs, with 4 fatalities occurring among 1,001 people experiencing anaphylactic reactions."*

'Pain' Adverse Drug Reactions: 157,579 events (4 fatal)

- *"A large number of these were arthralgias (joint pains – 24,902 ADRs) and myalgias (muscle pains – 31,168 ADRs), including fibromyalgia (270 ADRs)".*
- *"The head was the most common location for pain, but abdominal pain, eye pain, chest pain, pain in extremities, and anywhere else that pain can be imagined was reported. Headaches were reported more than 90,000 times and were associated with death in four people."*

Neurological Adverse Drug Reactions: 185,474 events (186 fatal)

- *"A wide variety of neurological ADRs were noted, including 1,992 ADRs involving seizures and 2,357 ADRs involving some form of paralysis, including Bell's palsy (626 ADRs). Other ADRs involving encephalopathy (18), dementia (33), ataxia [loss of balance, coordination, or speech] (34), spinal muscular atrophy (1), Parkinson's (18) and delirium (504) may reflect post-vaccination and neurodegenerative pathology."*
- *"The majority of fatalities associated with Nervous System ADRs occurred as a result of central nervous system hemorrhages"*
- *"More information is needed to determine the extent of the morbidity associated with this alarmingly large category of ADRs"*

Adverse Drug Reactions Involving Loss of Sight, Hearing, Speech, or Smell: 4,771 events

- *"There were 4,771 reports of visual impairment including blindness, 130 reports of speech impairment, 4,108 reports of taste impairment, 354 reports of olfactory impairment, and 704 reports of hearing impairment."*

Pregnancy Adverse Drug Reactions: 307 events (164 fatal)

- *"Given that vaccinated pregnant women comprise a small proportion of the vaccinated population in the UK up to 26th May 2021, there appear to be a high number of Pregnancy ADRs (307 ADRs), including one maternal death, 12 stillbirths (reported as 6 stillbirths and 6 fetal deaths, but only 3 listed as fatal(?)), one newborn death following preterm birth, and 150 spontaneous abortions."*

Here is the summary of all this information expressed as the Vegas odds of death and/or injury:

Calculating the Vegas Odds for the Vaccines (Yellow Card system - UK)

Adverse Event	Total	Fatal
Bleeding, Clotting and Ischaemic (Heart) Reactions	13,766	856
Immune System Adverse Drug Reactions	54,870	171
Pain' Adverse Drug Reactions	157,579	4
Neurological Adverse Drug Reactions	185,474	59
Adverse Drug Reactions involving sight, hearing, speech, smel	4,771	
Pregnancy Adverse Reactions	307	164

Total number of doses:	63,000,000
Total individual reports of adverse reactions	256,224
Total deaths:	1,253

	Death Only	Death or Adverse Drug Reaction
Vegas Odds	**1 : 50,279**	**1 : 246**

* Because the long-term trials are not complete, this chart only shows the odds for the KNOWN RISKS
Long-term risks are therefore impossible to quantify. Please factor this into your personal risk assessment.
*All data from the **UK's Yellow Card reporting system**, as aggregated by **Dr. Tess Lawrie***
*of **Evidence-based Medicine Consultancy Ltd***

https://b3d2650e-e929-4448-a527-4eeb59304c7f.filesusr.com/ugd/593c4f_b2acdef3774b4e9ca06e9fae526fd5cd.pdf

Figure 64: Data source: report published on June 9th by the Evidence-based Medicine Consultancy Ltd (Lawrie, 2021).

Clearly not all of the injuries will be severe or life-threatening. The UK numbers don't allow us to gauge what portion of those injuries are severe, but the data provided by the VAERS (Vaccine Adverse Event Reporting System) system maintained by the US CDC does provide this insight. Comparing the US numbers to the UK numbers also allows us to test if the vaccine reporting systems are consistent or wildly different from one country to the next. Consistent results are an indication that we are getting a reliable picture to help us assess our risks, whereas inconsistent results are a warning that we do not have a reliable picture of our risks.

So, here are the Vegas odds using data from the US VAERS system for deaths, all injuries, and only those injuries that the CDC categorized as severe:

Calculating the Vegas Odds for the Vaccines (CDC's VAERS system - USA)

Total number of doses:		313,034,386
Total adverse events:		324,562
Total adverse events (marked as "severe" only)		49,358
Total deaths:		5,165

	Death Only	Death or Severe Adverse Reaction	Any reaction
Vegas Odds	1 : 60,607	1 : 6,342	1 : 964

* Because the long-term trials are not complete, this chart only shows the odds for the KNOWN RISKS Long-term risks are therefore impossible to quantify. Please factor this into your personal risk assessment. All data from the US CDC's VAERS system (June 9th search). Bear in mind, VAERS is known to underreport, especially among less severe reactions.

https://wonder.cdc.gov/vaers.html

Figure 65: Data source: VAERS, June 9th search results for all reactions and filtered as "severe" only (CDC VAERS Query on June 9th, 2021).

It is important to point out that the odds shown in the previous chart are from a single dose. Although a number of health experts have stated that the risk of injury from the second dose is worse than the first, assuming that the risk remains the same from one dose to the next, the cumulative odds (using the US data) of two doses are:

- Death: 1 : 30,303
- Death or Severe Adverse Reaction: 1 : 3,171
- Any reaction: 1 : 482

And if people get a booster shot after 12 months, the cumulative odds after the third dose look like this:

- Death: 1 : 20,202
- Death or Severe Adverse Reaction: 1 : 2,114
- Any reaction: 1 : 321

And those cumulative odds keep adjusting for every subsequent booster shot.

25 — Vegas Odds Discussion

George Washington's soldiers knew their odds well. They could make an informed decision. When it comes to COVID, it is not so easy. Let's put some of these numbers in context.

Once more, for your benefit, I have reproduced the preliminary odds calculations of death from an infection with the virus in figure 66 along with the odds of death or injury caused by the vaccine in figure 67:

Calculating the Vegas Odds of Death from COVID, by Age Group

Age Groups SPLIT	0-17 (without pre-existing health conditions)	0-17 (with pre-existing health conditions)	18-49 (without pre-existing health conditions)	18-49 (with pre-existing health conditions)	50-64 (without pre-existing health conditions)	50-64 (with pre-existing health conditions)	+65 (without pre-existing health conditions)	+65 (with pre-existing health conditions)
Vegas Odds	zero risk	1 : 4,722	zero risk	1 : 500	1 : 1,683	1 : 122	1 : 28	1 : 14

Figure 66: The Vegas Odds of Death from COVID, by Age Group (summary of results from figure 61 above)

Calculating the Vegas Odds for the Vaccines (CDC's VAERS system - USA)

Total number of doses: 313,034,386
Total adverse events: 324,562
Total adverse events (marked as "severe" only) 49,358
Total deaths: 5,165

	Death Only	Death or Severe Adverse Reaction	Any reaction
Single Dose:	1 : 60,607	1 : 6,342	1 : 964
Two-dose:	1 : 30,303	1 : 3,171	1 : 482
Two-dose + 1 booster:	1 : 20,202	1 : 2,114	1 : 321

*Because the long-term trials are not complete, this chart only shows the odds for the KNOWN RISKS Long-term risks are therefore impossible to quantify. Please factor this into your personal risk assessment. All data from the **US CDC's VAERS system** (June 9th search). Bear in mind, VAERS is known to underreport, especially among less severe reactions.*

https://wonder.cdc.gov/vaers.html

Figure 67: Data source: VAERS, June 9th search results for all reactions and filtered as "severe" only (CDC VAERS Query on June 9th, 2021).

As these numbers show, anyone under the age of 49 who does not have pre-existing health conditions faces almost ZERO risk of death from COVID. For this group of people (along with anyone who has already been infected with SARS-CoV-2 and has recovered), the risk of death from the vaccine is clearly higher than the risk of death from the virus itself. They have nothing to gain and only something to lose from vaccination.

Everyone else has some risk of death from an infection with the virus, from as little at 1 in 4,722 for young people with pre-existing health conditions all the way up to 1 to 14 odds for someone 65 or older who is living with pre-existing health conditions.

To put these numbers in context, let's compare them to the odds of death if you are infected with some of the other dangerous diseases that we routinely vaccinate against:

- Measles will hospitalize 1 in 4 of those who catch it. It will kill anywhere between 0.1% and 25% of everyone that is infected (up to 1 million new deaths per year, every year) and often leaves survivors with severe life-long disabilities. It is the single leading cause of blindness in children in low-income countries (15,000 to 60,000 new cases per year) (Semba, 2004).

- Tetanus has a case fatality rate ranging from 10% to 80% in unvaccinated individuals.

- Diphtheria has a death rate of around 5-10%. For children under the age of 5 and for adults over the age of 40 the death rate rises to 20%.

- The death rate for meningitis can be as high as 70% and 1 in 5 survivors will be left with serious lifelong debilitating side effects like hearing loss, neurological damage, or an amputated limb.

As you can see, these diseases are in a completely different league than COVID, except for the very old living with severe pre-existing conditions. For them, COVID approaches the bottom end of risk level posed by some of these other deadly diseases.

But another difference between these other diseases and COVID is that, unless you are vaccinated, these other diseases pose a lifelong risk because you start being vulnerable the moment you are born, and you never stop being vulnerable until the day you die (unless you get immunity through disease or vaccination). COVID is a statistical nothingburger for those who are young, and only gets risky as you reach end of life.

Also, when it comes to these other deadly diseases, there is no cross-reactive immunity to be inherited from catching their closely related "cousins" because there aren't any less risky cousins floating around to offer you a lower-risk path to safety. With COVID there is.

As to the Vegas odds of the vaccines: the risk from the COVID vaccines is essentially impossible to quantify. The risk of death immediately after vaccination is reasonably consistent: 1 in 50,000 (UK) versus 1 in 60,000 (US) - these odds are in the same ballpark.

But we simply don't know the long-term risk associated with these vaccines because the long-term trials won't finish until 2024. Your long-term risk is a complete blind gamble, a shot in the dark. You literally have no idea what you are signing up for.

Furthermore, the range of serious and life-threatening conditions being reported are deeply alarming. These are more than just a mild temporary headache or a sore arm. How many of these injuries will result in permanent life-changing consequences? I don't know. How many will leave their victim vulnerable to developing other future medical conditions? I don't know, but considering the range and severity of these reactions, I am not sure I would want to be the guinea pig that finds out.

And some of the most alarming predictions made by critics, many of whom are widely cited doctors and researchers with long and distinguished careers, suggest that my attempt to calculate the Vegas odds for the vaccines does not capture anywhere near the full range of possible bad outcomes. How do you quantify the potential concerns they raise of leaky vaccines causing *antibody-dependent enhancement* (Wikipedia, n.d.) and mass-vaccination leading to more dangerous variants)? These critics may be wrong. But there is no data that can conclusively rule out their concerns. Time will tell. The most important test will come this winter when coronavirus seasonality puts our vaccinated friends to the test - that's when we will really find out whether all the concerns about things like antibody-dependent have merit or not.

If the critics are right, then those who have been vaccinated will have had their odds of death significantly increased when they next encounter a COVID virus in the wild. I hope with all my heart that the critics are wrong. Hope is not a strategy. A mass vaccine rollout with these kinds of overhanging questions is gross negligence on a scale never seen before.

I can understand why someone living in a nursing home with severe life-threatening pre-existing conditions might want to play the odds. I don't think I personally would, even then, but I also do not judge those who choose to go down that path. But I find it utterly reckless that the vaccine is being offered to anyone other than the most vulnerable among us, given the wide range of unknowns and the possible life-changing consequences of drawing the short straw in this gamble.

Asking someone to risk their life on vaccination in order to keep someone else safe is unethical. Even more so when those asked to take the risk cannot quantify their risk because the long-term risks of the vaccine remain unknown. Even more so when a large portion of the population that is being asked to take it has zero statistical risk of death from the virus itself. And even more so when coercion and misinformation is being used to strong-arm people into taking it.

For those under the age of 45 without pre-existing health conditions, for those with pre-existing cross-reactive immunity, and for those who have already had a COVID infection and/or have antibodies against the SARS-CoV-2 virus, there is no excuse whatsoever why they should be asked to risk their life on vaccination without any conceivable personal benefit to themselves.

But where does that leave the vulnerable? Doesn't that leave them without a ring of immunity and at risk from COVID? Let me show you how the concept of herd immunity is being willfully distorted to shame you into getting the jab.

26 — Protecting Babies in Cradles by Vaccinating Those Around Them

George Washington's ability to protect vulnerable babies in their cradles by vaccinating his troops illustrates the concept of herd immunity. By drying up the spread of the virus among his troops he also made the cradles in the villages in his path a much safer place to be. Not everyone is capable of getting vaccinated. Not everyone is capable of acquiring individual protection. Herd immunity, either acquired through natural exposure to a virus or through vaccination, creates a ring of immunity around the vulnerable.

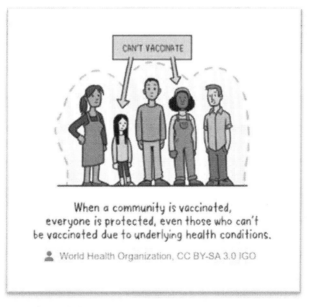

Figure 68: World Health Organization cartoon.

The idea of herd immunity doesn't apply to every disease. In the case of bacteria like tetanus, herd immunity is irrelevant because there is no person-to-person spread. The bacteria are waiting on the end of a rusty nail. The only form of protection that matters against tetanus is individual immunization.

Most other deadly diseases that we vaccinate against, like measles, rubella, meningitis, pertussis, tetanus, measles, diphtheria, chickenpox, and so on all depend on person-to-person transmission. Unlike COVID, many of these other diseases prey especially heavily on the young. Thus, many of those who face the highest risk from these other diseases are not capable of acquiring individual protection because they are either too young to get vaccinated or because they cannot get vaccinated while they are pregnant or immunocompromised. Ideally the latter categories already got immunized earlier in life (they had their chance to protect themselves before becoming vulnerable), but for the very young, until they reach the age that they can get vaccinated, their only means of protection against measles, mumps, meningitis, rubella, and so on is through the herd immunity of the community surrounding them.

COVID is unlike these diseases because once COVID vaccines became an option, the vulnerable stopped needing a ring of immunity because our health authorities have declared that they are all eligible to get individual protection from the jab.

27 — You Don't Need a Knight in Shining Armor to Ride to Granny's Rescue When She Can Have Her Own Sherman Tank

Before the emergency-use authorized COVID vaccines became available, lockdowns slowed spread among the healthy and therefore prevented a ring of herd immunity from forming around the vulnerable. At that time, the vulnerable desperately needed a ring of immunity because it was their only defense against the virus. Had the WHO's pandemic planning guidelines (WHO, 2019) been followed, the vulnerable would have been given focused protection while healthy members of the community would have continued living their lives unmolested by the government. In doing so, the healthy would have achieved natural herd immunity in 6 to 8 weeks, plus or minus, as happens every winter during flu season, after which the vulnerable would have been able to rejoin the community. Instead, they have been stuck behind bolted doors for a year and a half, at risk of everyone they meet.

But once vaccines became available that calculus changed. COVID is not a dangerous childhood disease that preys on newborns who cannot get vaccinated. The vulnerable during this pandemic are predominantly people with severe pre-existing health conditions. And according to our health officials, they are all now eligible for vaccination. They can all now acquire *individual* protection. Consequently, the herd immunity argument no longer applies.

The vaccine is being rolled out to the elderly, including long-term care patients with only a few months left to live. It is being rolled out to pregnant women. It is being rolled out to cancer patients prior to going into surgery or starting chemotherapy. It is being rolled out to people living with HIV and other immunocompromising conditions. Everyone now has the option of vaccination. Everyone who is vulnerable can get personal *individual* protection against COVID, if they want it. We no longer need to worry about trying to create a ring of immunity around the vulnerable because they now have the option to pop down to a clinic and acquire individual protection via the jab.

Protecting granny by getting the vaccine sounds like a noble cause. The dragon-slaying knight in shining armor, altruistically risking death from a vaccine by riding to granny's rescue to protect her from the COVID dragon. How virtuous, how honorable, and how utterly silly. Because if the vaccines work, granny now has the option to own her own dragon-slaying Sherman tank, complete with canon and bunker-busting dragon-killing rounds. And using coercion, like lies and vaccine passports, to force someone else to ride to granny's rescue is not just silly, it is a violation of all the principles that make us a free society.

The time for bravery and virtue was before vaccines became available. What was needed a year and a half ago was the courage of the healthy members of society to stand up to their fears and keep living their life so that a ring of immunity could have formed around granny. Now granny doesn't care what you do because she can get her own fully loaded tank with cup holders, a make-up mirror, and COVID-seeking missiles.

If the vaccine works, there is no case to be made for mass vaccination because the vulnerable can get the jab. But if vaccines don't work or if they are too risky, then we are right back where we started a year and a half ago when our only option to protect the vulnerable was to provide focused protection for the vulnerable while allowing the rest of society to acquire natural immunity to create a ring of immunity around the vulnerable.

28 — The Gamble…. Summary

So, let's return to that nasty tangled packet of lies that is being used to try to shame us into getting the jab: *"It's not about you, it is about saving lives by building a ring of immunity around the vulnerable to reduce the chance that they get infected."* No, it's 100% about you because you are the one taking the risk on the vaccine. And no, it is not about making a sacrifice to build a ring of immunity around the vulnerable because every single vulnerable individual now has the option of getting the jab.

Whether the vulnerable should take the risk of getting the emergency-use authorized vaccine is another question altogether. As I have demonstrated over the course of these pages, it is virtually impossible for anyone, regardless of age or underlying medical conditions, to give informed consent for the COVID vaccines because of how badly the government has distorted everyone's sense of risk. A sober look at the odds shows that the known risks of getting the jab are *no small matter* and that the unknown and unquantifiable risks hanging over this vaccine have turned what should be a basic risk calculation into a blind gamble.

George Washington took calculated risks. I do not think he would have approved of a gamble that asks those who are not vulnerable (and have little or nothing to personally gain from a COVID vaccination) to risk their lives on a vaccine with a sketchy risk profile and unquantifiable long-term risks, and to do all that in order to create a ring of immunity around those who no longer need a ring of immunity because they can protect themselves by getting the vax.

PART III —
The Snake-Oil Salesmen and the Covid-Zero Con: A Classic Bait-And-Switch for a Lifetime of Booster Shots (Immunity as a Service)

If a plumber with a lifetime of experience were to tell you that water runs uphill, you would know he is lying and that the lie is not accidental. It is a lie with a purpose. If you can also demonstrate that the plumber knows in advance that the product he is promoting with that lie is snake oil, you have evidence for a deliberate con. And once you understand what's really inside that bottle of snake oil, you will begin to understand the purpose of the con.

One of the most common reasons given for mass COVID vaccinations is the idea that if we reach herd immunity through vaccination, we can starve the virus out of existence and get our lives back. It's the COVID-Zero strategy or some variant of it.

By now it is abundantly clear from the epidemiological data that the vaccinated are able to both catch and spread the disease. Clearly vaccination isn't going to make this virus disappear. Only a mind that has lost its grasp on reality can fail to see how ridiculous all this has become.

But a tour through pre-COVID science demonstrates that, from day one, long before you and I had even heard of this virus, *it was 100% inevitable and 100% predictable* that these vaccines would never be capable of eradicating this coronavirus and would never lead to any kind of lasting herd immunity. Even worse, lockdowns and mass vaccination have created a dangerous set of circumstances that interfere with our immune system's ability to protect us against other respiratory viruses. They also risk driving the evolution of this virus towards mutations that are more dangerous to both the vaccinated and the unvaccinated alike. Lockdowns, mass vaccinations, and mass booster shots were never capable of delivering on any of the promises that were made to the public.

And yet, vaccination has been successfully used to control measles and even to eradicate smallpox. So, why not COVID? Immunity is immunity, and a virus is a virus is a virus, right? Wrong! Reality is far more complicated... and more interesting.

This Deep Dive exposes why, from day one, the promise of COVID-Zero can only ever have been a deliberately dishonest shell game designed to prey on a lack of public understanding of how our immune systems work and on how most respiratory viruses differ from other viruses that we routinely vaccinate against. We have been sold a fantasy designed to rope us into a pharmaceutical dependency as a deceitful trade-off for access to our lives. Variant by variant. For as long as the public is willing to go along for the ride.

Exposing this story does not require incriminating emails or whistleblower testimony. The story tells itself by diving into the long-established science that every single virologist, immunologist, evolutionary biologist, vaccine developer, and public health official had access to long before COVID began. As is so often the case, the devil is hidden in the details. As this story unfolds it will become clear that the one-two punch of lockdowns and the promise of vaccines as an exit strategy began as a cynical marketing ploy to coerce us into a never-ending regimen of annual booster shots intentionally designed to replace the natural "antivirus security updates" against respiratory viruses that come from hugs and handshakes and from children laughing together at school. We are being played for fools.

This is not to say that there aren't plenty of other opportunists taking advantage of this crisis to pursue other agendas and to tip society into a full-blown police state. One thing quickly morphs into another, and opportunists abound. But over the coming pages I will demonstrate that never-ending boosters (and the passports designed to enforce compliance) were the initial motive for this global social-engineering shell game — the subscription-based business model, adapted to the pharmaceutical industry. "Immunity as a service".

So, let's dive into the fascinating world of immune systems, viruses, and vaccines, layer by layer, to dispel the myths and false expectations that have been created by deceitful public health officials, pharmaceutical lobbyists, and media manipulators. What emerges as the lies are peeled apart is both surprising and more than a little alarming.

> *"Once you eliminate the impossible, whatever remains, no matter how improbable, must be the truth." - Sherlock Homes"* — Sir Arthur Conan Doyle

29 — Viral Reservoirs: The Fantasy of Eradication

Eradication of a killer virus sounds like a noble goal. In some cases it is, such as in the case of the smallpox virus. By 1980 we stopped vaccinating against smallpox because, thanks to widespread immunization, we starved the virus of available hosts for so long that it died out. No-one will need to risk their life on the side effects of a smallpox vaccination ever again because the virus is gone. It is a public health success story. Polio will hopefully be next — we're getting close.

But smallpox is one of only two viruses (along with rinderpest) that have been eradicated thanks to vaccination. Very few diseases meet the necessary criteria (Russell, 2011). Eradication is hard and only appropriate for very specific families of viruses.

Smallpox made sense for eradication because it was a uniquely human virus — there was no animal reservoir. By contrast, most respiratory viruses including SARS-CoV-2 (a.k.a. COVID) come from animal reservoirs: swine, birds, bats, etc. As long as there are bats in caves, birds in ponds, pigs in mud baths, and deer living in forests, respiratory viruses are only controllable through individual immunity, but it is not possible to eradicate them. There will always be a near-identical cousin brewing in the wings.

Even the current strain of COVID is already cheerfully jumping onwards across species boundaries. According to articles published by both *National Geographic* (National Geographic, August 2, 2021) and Nature magazine (Nature, August 2, 2021), 40% of wild deer tested positive for COVID antibodies in a study conducted in Michigan, Illinois, New York, and Pennsylvania. It has also been documented in wild mink (Nature, August 2, 2021) and has already made the species jump to other captive animals including dogs, cats, otters, leopards, tigers, and gorillas. A lot of viruses are not fussy. They happily adapt to new opportunities. Specialists, like smallpox, eventually go extinct. Generalists, like most respiratory viruses, never run out of hosts to keep the infection cycle going, forever.

As long as we share this planet with other animals, it is extremely deceitful to give anyone the impression that we can pursue any scorched earth policy that can put this genie back in the bottle. With an outbreak on this global scale, it was clear that we were always going to have to live with this virus. There are over 200 other endemic respiratory viruses that cause colds and flus, many of which circulate freely between humans and other animals. Now there are 201. They will be with us forever, whether we like it or not.

30 — SARS: The Exception to the Rule?

This all sounds well and good, but the original SARS virus did disappear, with public health measures like contact tracing and strict quarantine measures taking the credit. However, SARS was the exception to the rule. When it made the species jump to humans, it was so poorly adapted to its new human hosts that it had terrible difficulty spreading. This very poor level of adaptation gave SARS a rather unique combination of properties (BBC, September 28, 2020):

- SARS was extremely difficult to catch (it was never very contagious)
- SARS made people extremely sick.
- SARS did not have pre-symptomatic spread.

These three conditions made the SARS outbreak easy to control through contact tracing and through the quarantine of symptomatic individuals. SARS therefore never reached the point where it circulated widely among asymptomatic community members.

By contrast, by January/February of 2020 it was clear from experiences in China, Italy, and the outbreak on the *Diamond Princess* cruise ship (more on that story later) that the unique combination of conditions that made SARS controllable were not going to be the case with COVID. COVID was quite contagious (its rapid spread showed that COVID was already well adapted to spreading easily among its new human hosts), most people would have mild or no symptoms from COVID (making containment impossible), and that it was spreading by aerosols produced by both symptomatic and *pre-symptomatic* people (making contact tracing a joke).

In other words, it was clear by January/February 2020 that this pandemic would follow the normal rules of a *readily transmissible* respiratory epidemic (WHO, 2019), which cannot be reined in the way SARS was. Thus, by January/February of 2020, giving the public the impression that the SARS experience could be replicated for COVID was a deliberate lie - this genie was never going back inside the bottle.

31 — Fast Mutations: The Fantasy of Control Through Herd Immunity

Once a reasonably contagious respiratory virus begins circulating widely in a community, herd immunity can never be maintained for very long. RNA respiratory viruses (such as influenza viruses, respiratory syncytial virus (RSV) (Wikipedia, n.d.), rhinoviruses, and coronaviruses) all mutate extremely fast compared to viruses like smallpox, measles, or polio. Understanding the difference between something like measles and a virus like COVID is key to understanding the con that is being perpetrated by our health institutions. Bear with me here, I promise not to get too technical.

All viruses survive by creating copies of themselves. And there are always a lot of "imperfect copies" — mutations — produced by the copying process itself. Among RNA respiratory viruses these mutations stack up so quickly that there is rapid genetic drift, which continually produces new strains. Variants are normal. Variants are expected. Variants make it virtually impossible to build the impenetrable wall of long-lasting herd immunity required to starve these respiratory viruses out of existence. That's one of several reasons why flu vaccines don't provide long-lasting immunity and have to be repeated annually — our immune system constantly needs to be updated to keep pace with the inevitable evolution of countless unnamed "variants."

This never-ending conveyor belt of mutations means that everyone's immunity to COVID was always only going to be temporary and only offer partial cross-reactive protection against future re-infections. Thus, from day one, COVID vaccination was always doomed to the same fate as the flu vaccine — a lifelong regimen of annual booster shots to try to keep pace with "variants" for those unwilling to expose themselves to the risk of a natural infection. And the hope that by the time the vaccines (and their booster shots) roll off the production line, they won't already be out of date when confronted by the current generation of virus mutations.

Genetic drift caused by mutations is *much* slower in viruses like measles, polio, or smallpox, which is why herd immunity can be used to control these other viruses (or even eradicate them as in the case of smallpox or polio). The reason that the common respiratory viruses have such rapid genetic drift compared to these other viruses has much less to do with how many errors are produced during the copying process and much more to do with how many of those "imperfect" copies are actually able to survive and produce more copies (Science Daily, May 21, 2015).

A simple virus with an uncomplicated attack strategy for taking over host cells can tolerate a lot more mutations than a complex virus with a complicated attack strategy. Complexity and specialization put limits on how many of those imperfect copies have a chance at becoming successful mutations. Simple machinery doesn't break down as easily if there is an imperfection in the mechanical parts. Complicated high-tech machinery will not work if there are even minor flaws in precision parts.

For example, before a virus can hijack the DNA of a host cell to begin making copies of itself, the virus needs to unlock the cell wall to gain entry. Cellular walls are made of proteins and are coated by sugars; viruses need to find a way to create a doorway through that protein wall. A virus like influenza uses a very simple strategy to get inside — it locks onto one of the sugars on the outside of the cell wall in order to piggyback a ride when the sugar molecule is absorbed into the cell (cells use sugar as their energy source). It's such a simple strategy that it allows the influenza virus to go through lots of mutations without losing its ability to gain entry to the cell. Influenza's simplicity makes it very adaptable and allows many different types of mutations to thrive as long as they all use the same piggyback entry strategy to get inside host cells.

By contrast, something like the measles virus uses a highly specialized and very complicated strategy to gain entry to a host cell. It relies on very specialized surface proteins to break open a doorway into the host cell. It's a very rigid and complex system that doesn't leave a lot of room for errors in the copying process. Even minor mutations to the measles virus will cause changes to its surface proteins, leaving it unable to gain access to a host cell to make more copies of itself. Thus, even if there are lots of mutations, those mutations are almost all evolutionary dead ends, thus preventing genetic drift. That's one of several reasons why both a natural infection and vaccination against measles creates lifetime immunity — immunity lasts because new variations don't change much over time.

Most RNA respiratory viruses have a high rate of genetic drift because they all rely on relatively simple attack strategies to gain entry to host cells. This allows mutations to stack up quickly without becoming evolutionary dead ends because they avoid the evolutionary trap of complexity.

Coronaviruses use a different strategy than influenza to gain access to host cells. They have proteins on the virus surface (the infamous S-spike protein, the same one that is mimicked by the vaccine injection), which latches onto a receptor on the cell surface (the ACE2 receptor) — a kind of key to unlock the door. This attack strategy is a little bit more complicated than the system used by influenza, which is probably why genetic drift in coronaviruses is slightly slower than in influenza, but it is still a much much simpler and much less specialized system than the one used by measles. Coronaviruses, like other respiratory viruses, are therefore constantly producing a never-ending conveyor belt of "variants" that make long-lasting herd immunity impossible. Variants are normal. The alarm raised by our public health authorities about "variants" and the feigned compassion of pharmaceutical companies as they rush to develop fresh boosters capable of fighting variants is a charade, much like expressing surprise about the sun rising in the East.

Once you got immunity to smallpox, measles, or polio, you had full protection for a few decades and were protected against severe illness or death for the rest of your life. But for fast-mutating respiratory viruses, including coronaviruses, within a few months they are sufficiently different that your previously acquired immunity will only ever offer *partial* protection against your next exposure. The fast rate of mutation ensures that you never catch the exact same cold or flu twice, just their closely related constantly evolving cousins. What keeps you from feeling the full brunt of each new infection is *cross-reactive immunity*, which is another part of the story of how you are being conned, which I will come back to shortly.

32 — Blind Faith in Central Planning: The Fantasy of Timely Doses

But let's pretend for a moment that a miraculous vaccine could be developed that could give us all 100% sterilizing immunity today. The length of time it takes to manufacture and ship 8 billion doses (and then make vaccination appointments for 8 billion people) ensures that by the time the last person gets their last dose, the never-ending conveyor belt of mutations will have already rendered the vaccine partially ineffective. True sterilizing immunity simply won't ever happen with coronaviruses. The logistics of rolling out vaccines to 8 billion people meant that none of our vaccine makers or public health authorities ever could have genuinely believed that vaccines would create lasting herd immunity against COVID.

So, for a multitude of reasons, it was a deliberate lie to give the public the impression that if enough people take the vaccine, it would create lasting herd immunity. It was 100% certain, from day one, that by the time the last dose is administered, the rapid evolution of the virus would ensure that it would already be time to start thinking about booster shots. Exactly like the flu shot. Exactly the opposite of a measles vaccine. Vaccines against respiratory viruses can *never* provide anything more than a temporary *cross-reactive immunity "update"* — they are merely a synthetic replacement for your annual natural exposure to the smorgasbord of cold and flu viruses. Immunity as a service, imposed on society by trickery. The only question was always, how long between booster shots? Weeks, months, years? Feeling conned yet?

33 — Spiked: The Fantasy of Preventing Infection

The current crop of COVID vaccines was never designed to provide sterilizing immunity - that's not how they work. They are merely a tool designed to teach the immune system to attack the S-spike protein, thereby priming the immune system to reduce the *severity* of infection in preparation for your inevitable future encounter with the real virus. They were never capable of preventing infection, nor of preventing spread. They were merely designed to reduce your chance of being hospitalized or dying if you are infected. As former FDA commissioner Scott Gottlieb, who is on Pfizer's board, said: "*the original premise behind these vaccines were [sic] that they would substantially reduce the risk of death and severe disease and hospitalization. And that was the data that came out of the initial clinical trials.*" (The British Medical Journal, August 23, 2021) Every first-year medical student knows that you cannot get herd immunity from a vaccine that does not stop infection.

In other words, by their design, these vaccines can neither stop you from catching an infection nor stop you from transmitting the infection to someone else. They were never capable of creating herd immunity. They were designed to protect individuals against severe outcomes if they choose to take them - a tool to provide temporary focused protection for the vulnerable, just like the flu vaccine. Pushing for mass vaccination was a con from day one. And the idea of using vaccine passports to separate the vaccinated from the unvaccinated was also a con from day one. The only impact these vaccine passports have on the pandemic is as a coercive tool to get you to roll up your sleeve. Nothing more.

34 — Antibodies, B-Cells, and T-Cells: Why Immunity to Respiratory Viruses Fades So Quickly

There are multiple interconnected parts to why immunity to COVID, or any other respiratory virus, is always only temporary. Not only is the virus constantly mutating but immunity itself fades over time, not unlike the way our brains start forgetting how to do complicated math problems unless they keep practicing. This is true for both immunity acquired through natural infection and immunity acquired through vaccination.

Our immune systems have a kind of immunological memory — basically, how long does your immune system remember how to launch an attack against a specific kind of threat. That memory fades over time. For some vaccines, like diphtheria and tetanus, that immunological memory fades *very* slowly. The measles vaccine protects for life. But for others, like the flu vaccine, that immunological memory faces very quickly.

On average, the flu vaccine is only about 40% effective to begin with. And it begins to fade almost immediately after vaccination. By about 150 days (5 months), it reaches zero.

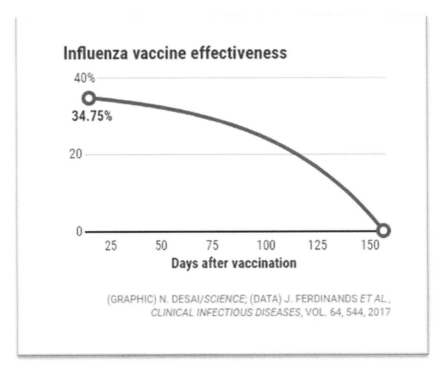

Figure 69: Fading immunity after the flu shot (Science, April 18th, 2019)

The solution to this strange phenomenon lies in the different types of immune system responses that are triggered by a vaccine (or by exposure to the real thing through a natural infection). This has big implications for coronavirus vaccines, but I'll get to that in a moment. First a little background information...

A good analogy is to think of our immune system like a medieval army. The first layer of protection began with generalists - guys armed with clubs that would take a swing at everything - they were good for keeping robbers and brigands at bay and for conducting small skirmishes. But if the attack was bigger, then these generalists were quickly overwhelmed, serving as arrow fodder to blunt the attack on the more specialized troops coming up behind them. Spearmen, swordsmen, archers, cavalry, catapult operators, siege tower engineers, and so on. Each additional layer of defense has a more expensive kit and takes ever greater amounts of time to train (an English longbowman took years to build up the necessary skill and strength to become effective). The more specialized a troop is, the more you want to hold them back from the fight unless it's absolutely necessary because they are expensive to train, expensive to deploy, and make a bigger mess when they fight, which needs to be cleaned up afterwards. Always keep your powder dry. Send in the arrow fodder first and slowly ramp up your efforts from there.

Our immune system relies on a similar kind of layered system of defense. In addition to various non-specific rapid response layers that take out the brigands, like natural killer cells, macrophages, mast cells, and so on, we also have many adaptive (specialized) layers of antibodies (i.e. IgA, IgG, IgM immunoglobulin) and various types of highly specialized white blood cells, like B-cells and T-cells. Some antibodies are released by regular B-cells. Others are released by blood plasma. Then there are memory B-cells, which are capable of remembering previous threats and creating new antibodies long after the original antibodies fade away. And there are various types of T-cells (again with various degrees of immunological memory), like natural killer T-cells, killer T-cells, and helper T-cells, all of which play various roles in detecting and neutralizing invaders. In short, the greater the threat, the more troops are called into the fight.

This is clearly a gross oversimplification of all the different interconnected parts of our immune system, but the point is that a mild infection doesn't trigger as many layers whereas a severe infection enlists the help of deeper layers, which are slower to respond but are much more specialized in their attack capabilities. And if those deeper adaptive layers get involved, they are capable of retaining a memory of the threat in order to be able to mount a quicker attack if a repeat attack is recognized in the future. That's why someone who was infected by the dangerous Spanish Flu in 1918 might still have measurable T-cell immunity a century later but the mild bout of winter flu you had a couple of years ago might not have triggered T-cell immunity, even though both may have been caused by versions of the same H1N1 influenza virus.

As a rule of thumb, the broader the immune response, the longer immunological memory will last. Antibodies fade in a matter of months, whereas B-cell and T-cell immunity can last a lifetime.

Another rule of thumb is that a higher viral load puts more strain on your immune defenses, thus overwhelming the rapid response layers and forcing the immune system to enlist the deeper adaptive layers. That's why nursing homes and hospitals are more dangerous places for vulnerable people than backyard barbeques. That's why feedlot cattle are more vulnerable to viral diseases than cattle on pasture. Viral load matters a lot to how easily the generalist layers are overwhelmed and how much effort your immune system has to make to neutralize a threat.

Where the infection happens in the body also matters. For example, an infection in the upper respiratory tract triggers much less involvement from your adaptive immune system than when it reaches your lungs. Part of this is because your upper respiratory tract is already heavily preloaded with large numbers of generalist immunological cells that are designed to attack germs as they enter, which is why most colds and flus never make it deeper into the lungs. The guys with the clubs are capable of handling most of the threats that try to make through the gate. Most of the specialized troops hold back unless they are needed.

Catching a dangerous disease like measles produces lifetime immunity because an infection triggers all the deep layers that will retain a memory of how to fight off future encounters with the virus. So does the measles vaccine. Catching a cold or mild flu generally does not.

From an evolutionary point of view, this actually makes a lot of sense. Why waste valuable resources developing long-lasting immunity (i.e. training archers and building catapults) to defend against a virus that did not put you in mortal danger. A far better evolutionary strategy is to evolve a narrower generalist immune response to mild infections (i.e. most cold and flu viruses), which fades quickly once the threat is conquered, but invest in deep long-term broad-based immunity to dangerous infections, which lasts a very long time in case that threat is ever spotted on the horizon again. Considering the huge number of threats our immune systems face, this strategy avoids the trap of spreading immunological memory too thin. Our immunological memory resources are not limitless - long-term survival requires prioritizing our immunological resources.

The take-home lesson is that vaccines will, at best, only last as long as immunity acquired through natural infection and will often fade much faster because the vaccine is often only able to trigger a partial immune response compared to the actual infection. So, if the disease itself doesn't produce a broad-based immune response leading to long-lasting immunity, neither will the vaccine. And in most cases, immunity acquired through vaccination will begin to fade much sooner than immunity acquired through a natural infection. Every vaccine maker and public health official knows this despite bizarrely claiming that the COVID vaccines (based on re-creating the S-protein spike instead of using a whole virus) would somehow become the exception to the rule (John Hopkins Bloomberg School of Public Health, May 28, 2021). That was a lie, and they knew it from day one. That should set your alarm bells ringing at full throttle.

So, with this little bit of background knowledge under our belts, let's look at what our public health officials and vaccine makers would have known in advance about coronaviruses and coronavirus vaccines when they told us back in the early Spring of 2020 that COVID vaccines were the path back to normality.

From a 2003 study (Holmes, 2003): "*Until SARS appeared, human coronaviruses were known as the cause of* **15–30% of colds**... *Colds are generally mild, self-limited infections, and significant increases in neutralizing antibody titer are found in nasal secretions and serum after infection. Nevertheless, some* **unlucky individuals can be reinfected with the same coronavirus soon after recovery and get symptoms again.**" [my emphasis]

In other words, the coronaviruses involved in colds (there were four human coronaviruses before SARS, MERS, and COVID) all trigger such a weak immune response that they do not lead to any long-lasting immunity whatsoever. And why would they if, for most of us, the threat is so minimal that the generalists are perfectly capable of neutralizing the attack.

We also know that immunity against coronaviruses is not durable in other animals either. As any farmer knows well, cycles of reinfection with coronaviruses are the rule rather than the exception among their livestock (for example, coronaviruses are a common cause of pneumonia and various types of diarrheal diseases like scours, shipping fever, and winter dysentery in cattle). Annual farm vaccination schedules are therefore designed accordingly. The lack of long-term immunity to coronaviruses is well documented in veterinary research (Saif, 2010) among cattle, poultry, deer, water buffalo, etc. Furthermore, although animal coronavirus vaccines have been on the market for many years, it is well known that "*none are completely efficacious in animals*" (Saif, 2020). So, like the fading flu vaccine profile I showed you earlier, none of the animal coronavirus vaccines are capable of providing sterilizing immunity (none were capable of stopping 100% of infections, without which you can never achieve long-lasting herd immunity) and the partial immunity they offered is well known to fade rather quickly.

What about immunity to COVID's close cousin, the deadly SARS coronavirus, which had an 11% case fatality rate during the 2003 outbreak? From a 2007 study (Wu et al., 2007): "*SARS-specific antibodies were maintained for an average of 2 years... SARS patients might be susceptible to reinfection >3 years after initial exposure.*" (Bear in mind that, as with all diseases, re-infection does not mean you are necessarily going to get full-blown SARS; fading immunity after a natural infection tends to offer at least some level of partial protection against severe outcomes for a considerable amount of time after you can already be reinfected and spread it to others - more on that later.)

And what about MERS, the deadliest coronavirus to date, which made the jump from camels in 2012 and had a fatality rate of around 35%? It triggered the broadest immune response (due to its severity) and also appears to trigger the longest lasting immunity as a result (> 6yrs (Alshukairi, 2021))

Thus, to pretend there was any chance that herd immunity to COVID would be anything but short-lived was dishonest at best. For most people, immunity was always going to fade quickly. Just like what happens after most other respiratory virus infections. By February 2020, the epidemiological data showed clearly that for most people COVID was a mild coronavirus (nowhere near as severe than SARS or MERS), so it was virtually a certainty that even the immunity from a natural infection would fade within months, not years. It was also a certainty that vaccination was therefore, at best, only ever going to provide partial protection and that this protection would be temporary, lasting on the order of months. This is a case of false and misleading advertising if there ever was one.

If I can allow my farming roots to shine through for a moment, I'd like to explain the implications of what was known about animal coronaviruses vaccines. Baby calves are often vaccinated against bovine coronaviral diarrhea shortly after birth if they are born in the spring mud and slush season, but not if they are born in midsummer on lush pastures where the risk of infection is lower. Likewise, bovine coronavirus vaccines are used to protect cattle before they face stressful conditions during shipping, in a feedlot, or in winter feed pens. Animal coronavirus vaccines are thus used as tools to provide a *temporary* boost in immunity, in very specific conditions, and only for very specific vulnerable categories of animals. After everything I've laid out so far in this text, the targeted use of bovine coronavirus vaccines (focused protection for the vulnerable) should surprise no-one. Pretending that our human coronavirus vaccines would be different was nonsense.

The only rational reason why the WHO and public health officials would withhold all that contextual information from the public as they rolled out lockdowns and held forth vaccines as an exit strategy was to whip the public into irrational fear in order to be able to make a dishonest case for mass vaccination when they should have, at most, been focused on providing focused vaccination of the most vulnerable only. That deception was the Trojan Horse to introduce endless mass booster shots as immunity inevitably fades and as new variants replace old ones.

Now, as all the inevitable limitations and problems with these vaccines become apparent (i.e. the rapid fade of vaccine-induced immunity, vaccines proving to only be partially effective, the rise of new variants, and the vaccinated population demonstrably catching and spreading the virus — a.k.a. the leaky vaccine phenomenon) (Swiss Policy Research, August 20, 2021), the surprise that our health authorities are showing simply isn't credible. As I have shown you, all this was 100% to be expected. They intentionally weaponized fear and false expectations to unleash a fraudulent bait-and-switch racket of global proportions. Immunity on demand, forever.

35 — Manufacturing Dangerous Variants: Lessons From the 1918 Spanish Flu

At this point you may be wondering, if there is no lasting immunity from infection or vaccination, then are public health officials right to roll out booster shots to protect us from severe outcomes even if their dishonest methods to get us to accept them were unethical? Do we need a lifetime regimen of booster shots to keep us safe from a beast to which we cannot develop durable long-term immunity?

The short answer is no.

Contrary to what you might think, the rapid evolution of RNA respiratory viruses actually has several important benefits for us as their involuntary hosts, which protect us without the benefit of broad lifelong immunity. One of those benefits has to do with the natural evolution of the virus towards less dangerous variants. The other is the cross-reactive immunity that comes from frequent re-exposure to closely related "cousins". I'm going to peel apart both of these topics in order to show you the remarkable system that nature designed to keep us safe... and to show you how the policies being forced on us by our public health authorities are knowingly interfering with this system. They are creating a dangerous situation that increases our risk to other respiratory viruses (not just to COVID) and may even push the COVID virus to evolve to become more dangerous to both the unvaccinated and the vaccinated. There are growing signs that this nightmare scenario has already begun (Swiss Policy Research, August 20, 2021).

"In this present crisis, government is not the solution to our problem; government is the problem." — President Ronald Reagan in 1981.

Let's start with the evolutionary pressures that normally drive viruses towards becoming less dangerous over time. A virus depends on its host to spread it. A lively host is more useful than a bedridden or dead one because a lively host can spread the virus further and will still be around to catch future mutations. Viruses risk becoming evolutionary dead ends if they kill or immobilize their hosts. Plagues came, killed, and then were starved out of existence because their surviving hosts all acquired herd immunity. Colds come and go every year because their hosts are lively, easily spread the viruses around, and never acquire long-lasting immunity so that last year's hosts can also serve as next year's hosts — only those who have weak immune systems have much to worry about. In other words, under normal conditions, mutations that are more contagious but less deadly have a survival advantage over less contagious and more deadly variations.

From the virus' point of view, the evolutionary golden mean is reached when it can easily infect as many hosts as possible without reducing their mobility and without triggering long-term immunity in most of their hosts. That's the ticket to setting up a sustainable cycle of reinfection, forever. Viruses with slow genetic drift and highly specialized reproductive strategies, like polio or measles, can take centuries or longer to become less deadly and more contagious; some may never reach the relatively harmless status of a cold or mild flu virus (by harmless I mean harmless to the majority of the population despite being extremely dangerous to those with weak or compromised immune systems). But for viruses with fast genetic drift, like respiratory viruses, even a few months can make a dramatic difference. Rapid genetic drift is one of the reasons why the Spanish Flu stopped being a monster disease, but polio and measles haven't. *And anyone with training in virology or immunology understands this!*

We often speak of evolutionary pressure as though it forces an organism to adapt. In reality, a simple organism like a virus is utterly blind to its environment — all it does is blindly produce genetic

190

copies of itself. "Evolutionary pressure" is actually just a fancy way of saying that environmental conditions will determine which of those millions of copies survives long enough to produce even more copies of itself.

A human adapts to its environment by altering its behavior (that's one type of adaptation). But the behavior of a single viral particle never changes. A virus "adapts" over time because some genetic copies with one set of mutations survive and spread faster than other copies with a different set of mutations. Adaptation in viruses has to be seen exclusively through the lens of changes from one generation of virus to the next based on which mutations have a competitive edge over others. And that competitive edge will vary depending on the kind of environmental conditions a virus encounters.

So, fear mongering about the Delta variant being even more contagious leaves out the fact that this is *exactly* what you would expect as a respiratory virus adapts to its new host species. We would expect new variants to be more contagious but less deadly as the virus fades to become just like the other 200+ respiratory viruses that cause common colds and flus.

That's also why the decision to lock down the healthy population is so sinister. Lockdowns, border closures, and social distancing rules reduced spread among the healthy population, thus creating a situation where mutations produced among the healthy would become sufficiently rare that they might be outnumbered by mutations circulating among the bedridden. Mutations circulating among the healthy are, by definition, going to be the least dangerous mutations since they did not make their hosts sick enough to confine them to bedrest. That's precisely the variants you want to spread in order to drown out competition from more dangerous mutations.

A host stuck in bed with a fever and not out dining with friends is limited in his ability to infect others compared to a host infected with a variety that only gives its host a sniffle. Not all bedridden hosts have caught a more dangerous mutation, but all dangerous mutations will be found among the bedridden. Thus, as time goes by, dangerous mutations can only compete with less dangerous mutations if the entire population is limited in its ability to mix and mingle.

As long as the majority of infections are among the healthy, the more dangerous variants circulating among some of the bedridden will be outnumbered and will become evolutionary dead ends. But when public health officials intentionally restricted spread among the young, strong, and healthy members of society by imposing lockdowns, they created a set of evolutionary conditions that risked shifting the competitive evolutionary advantage from the least dangerous variants to more dangerous variants. By locking us all up, they risked making the virus more dangerous over time. Evolution doesn't sit around to wait for you while you develop a vaccine.

Let me give you a historical example to demonstrate that this rapid evolution of a virus towards either more or less dangerous variants isn't mere theory. Small changes to the environment can lead to *very* rapid changes in the virus' evolution. The first wave of the 1918 Spanish Flu was not particularly deadly with mortality rates similar to regular seasonal flu (History Channel, December 22, 2020). However, the second wave was not only much deadlier but, rather unusually, was particularly deadly to young people rather than just the old and the weak. Why would the *second* wave be the deadly one? And what would cause the virus to evolve so quickly to become both more deadly and better adapted to preying on young people? At first glance it would seem to defy all evolutionary logic.

The answer demonstrates just how sensitive a virus is to small changes in evolutionary pressure. The Spanish Flu spread in the midst of the lockdown-mimicking conditions of World War One. During the first wave, the virus found a huge population of soldiers trapped in the cold damp conditions of the trenches and a near endless supply of captive bedridden hosts in overflowing field hospitals. By the Spring of 1918, up to three-quarters of the entire French military and half of British troops had been infected. These conditions created two unique evolutionary pressures. On the one hand, it allowed variants that were well adapted to young people to emerge. But on the other hand, unlike normal times, the cramped conditions of trench warfare and field hospitals allowed dangerous variants that immobilize their hosts to spread freely with little competition from less dangerous variants that spread through lively hosts. The trenches and field hospitals became the virus incubators driving the evolution of variants.

Normally young people are predominantly exposed to less dangerous mutations because the healthiest do all the mingling while the bedridden stay home. But the lockdown conditions of war created conditions that erased the competitive advantage of less dangerous mutations that don't immobilize their hosts, leading to the rise of more dangerous mutations.

Thanks to the end of the war, the lockdown-mimicking conditions also ended, thereby shifting the competitive advantage back to less dangerous mutations that could spread freely among the mobile healthy members of the population. The deadliness of the second wave of the 1918 Spanish Flu is inextricably linked to the First World War, and the end of the war is linked to the virus fading into the background of regular cold and flu season.

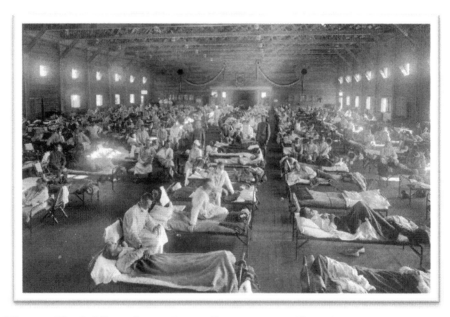

Figure 70: Soldiers from Fort Riley, Kansas, ill with Spanish flu at a hospital ward at Camp Funston

It is therefore highly likely that the 1918 Spanish Flu would never have been more than a really bad flu season had it not been for the amplifying effect of lockdown conditions created by a world at war.

It also raises the question, for which I don't have an answer, whether the lockdown strategy during COVID was *intentionally* used to reduce spread among the healthy in order to keep the virus from fading into harmless irrelevancy. I use the word "intentionally" — and it's a strong word — because the deadly second wave of the 1918 Spanish Flu and its causes are hardly secrets in the medical community. You'd have to be a completely reckless and utterly incompetent idiot, or a cynical bastard with an agenda, to impose any strategy that mimics those virus-amplifying conditions. Yet that's what our health authorities did. And what they continue to do while shamelessly hyperventilating about the risk of "variants" to force us to submit to medical tyranny based on mandatory vaccines, never-ending booster shots, and vaccine passports that can turn off access to our normal lives. This is cynicism at its finest.

36 — Leaky Vaccines, Antibody-Dependent Enhancement, and the Marek Effect

The experience of the 2nd wave of the 1918 Spanish Flu also raises another question: What kind of evolutionary pressures are being created by using a leaky vaccine?

A vaccine that provides *sterilizing* immunity prevents the vaccinated from being able to catch or transmit the virus. They become a dead end for the virus. However, as I've already mentioned, the current crop of COVID vaccines, which are meant to train the immune system to recognize the S-spike proteins, were not designed to create sterilizing immunity. By their design, they merely help reduce the risk of severe outcomes by priming the immune system. The vaccinated can still catch and spread the virus — the definition of a leaky vaccine — and epidemiological data makes it very clear that this is now happening all around the world. Thus, both the vaccinated and the unvaccinated are equally capable of producing new variants. The idea that the unvaccinated are producing variants while the vaccinated are not, is a boldfaced lie.

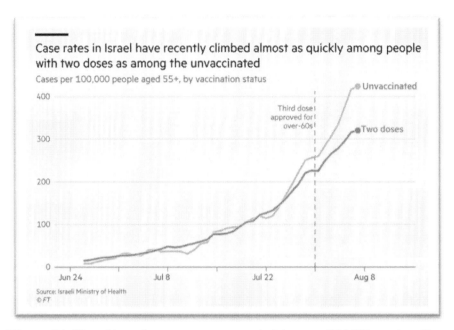

Figure 71: "*Israel hopes boosters can avert new lockdown as COVID vaccine efficacy fades.*" (Financial Times, August 23rd, 2021)

From an evolutionary perspective, this is a potentially dangerous scenario. What has been done by temporarily blunting the risk of hospitalization or death, but without stopping infection among the vaccinated, is to create a set of evolutionary conditions where a variant that is dangerous to the unvaccinated can spread easily among the vaccinated without making the vaccinated very sick. For lack of a better term, let's call this a dual-track variant. Thus, because the vaccinated are not getting bedridden from this dual-track variant, they can continue to spread it easily, giving it a competitive advantage, even if it is highly dangerous to the unvaccinated.

Furthermore, since COVID vaccination only offers temporary short-term protection, as soon as immunity fades the vaccinated themselves are also equally at risk of more severe outcomes. Thus, this creates the evolutionary pressure for the virus to behave as an increasingly contagious but relatively mild virus as long as everyone is vaccinated but as a dangerous but also very contagious virus as soon as temporary immunity wears off. The call for boosters every 6 months is already here (Wall Street Journal, August 26, 2021) (Update: now it's being revised down to 5 months. (Bloomberg, August 27, 2021))

So, the pandemic really does have the potential to become the *Pandemic of the Unvaccinated* (the shameless term coined by public health officials to terrify the vaccinated into bullying their unvaccinated peers), but reality comes with a twist because if a dual-track variant does evolve it would be the unvaccinated (and those whose boosters have expired) who would have reason to fear the vaccinated, not the other way around as so many frightened citizens seem to believe. And the end result would be that we all become permanently dependent on boosters every 6 months, forever.

Hold on, you might say, the flu vaccine chart shown earlier also never provided sterilizing immunity. The flu vaccine is notoriously leaky but hasn't gotten more dangerous, has it? The answer is complicated because the comparison is less useful than it first appears. As long as the majority of the population does not get the flu vaccine, more dangerous variants will face stiff competition from less dangerous ones circulating among the healthy unvaccinated population (average flu vaccination rates in most western countries are between 38-41% (American Council on Science and Health, October 26, 2018), with most other countries around the world doing very little vaccination against the flu). And since the vaccine is only 40% effective to begin with and since immunity fades rapidly after the shot, the flu vaccine doesn't provide much protection to begin with, thus reducing the chance that separate mutations would circulate among the vaccinated. And public health frequently gets the strain wrong (influenza has many strains that are constantly evolving so there is a lot of guesswork that goes into creating the right vaccine formula each year). In other words, lack of universal coverage and poor protection are likely preventing the emergence of a dual-track variant.

Furthermore, flu vaccination is not evenly distributed across the population. As long as flu vaccination is voluntary, it is mostly the vulnerable and those who work around them that get it while children, young adults and other healthy members of society don't get it. So, even if more deadly variants were to arise in nursing homes or hospital settings, the high number of healthy unvaccinated visitors to those facilities would constantly bring less deadly more contagious variants with them, thereby preventing more dangerous variants from gaining a competitive edge in nursing home or hospital settings. But if the leaky flu vaccinations were to be extended to everyone, or if nursing home populations continue to be kept isolated from the rest of society during COVID lockdowns, things might begin to look a little different.

However, what I am warning about is far from theoretical. There is a very clear example (well known to public health officials and vaccine developers) from the poultry farming industry where a universal leaky vaccine pushed a virus to evolve to become extremely deadly to unvaccinated chickens (PBS Science, July 27, 2015). It is called the Marek Effect (eugyppius, August 11, 2021). It began with a leaky vaccine that was rolled out to fight a herpes virus in industrialized high-density chicken barns. Vaccinated chickens were protected from severe outcomes but nevertheless continued to catch and spread the virus, so evolutionary pressure led to the emergence of a dual-track variant that become the dominant strain of this herpes virus. It continues to spread among the vaccinated chickens without killing them but kills up to 80% or more of unvaccinated birds if they get infected. Thus, a never-ending stream of vaccinations is now required just to maintain the status quo. I bet the pharmaceutical industry is smiling at all those drug-dependent chickens though — talk about having a captive audience!

It's not a certainty that this will happen with the COVID vaccines, but the longer this fiasco continues and the higher that vaccination rates rise around the world, the more likely it becomes that we re-create the conditions for some kind of Marek effect to develop. A leaky vaccine used sparingly to protect small pockets of vulnerable individuals is very different than a leaky vaccine applied to everyone.

The rapid change in behavior of the 1918 Spanish Flu should be a warning to us all that a virus can adapt very quickly in response to small changes in evolutionary pressure. The closer we get to universal vaccination, the greater the danger that leaky vaccines will lead to dual-track variants that become more dangerous to the unvaccinated.

There is one other danger from leaky vaccines that is worth mentioning because researchers are already starting to see the first signs of it, as you can see discussed in a paper published on August 9th, 2021, in the *Journal of Infection* (Yahi et al., August 9, 2021). It's called antibody-dependent enhancement (ADE) (Wikipedia, n.d.). It happens when a poorly designed vaccine trains antibodies to recognize a virus as an intruder without being strong enough to kill/neutralize them. Instead of the virus being neutralized inside the antibody when the antibody attacks and "swallows" the virus (antibodies envelope intruders in order to neutralize them), the virus takes over the antibody cell that attacked it and uses it as a host to start making copies of itself. Thus, the attacking antibody opens the door to the inside of the cell and becomes the virus' unwitting host, thereby accelerating rather than stopping the infection.

Antibody-dependent enhancement is a well-documented phenomenon in attempts to develop vaccines against the RSV virus, dengue fever, *and other coronaviruses* (Su et al., 2020) This is one of the reasons why previous attempts to develop a human coronavirus vaccine against the SARS virus failed. ADE kept happening in animal trials. And many doctors warned from day one that it would happen with these vaccines as well as new variants gradually emerge that are sufficiently different from the original variant upon which the vaccine is based. ADE doesn't show up on the day after vaccination. It emerges gradually as new variants spread that are different from previous variants.

This quote is from the aforementioned study (Su et al., 2020): "*ADE may be a concern for people receiving vaccines based on the original Wuhan strain spike sequence (either mRNA or viral vectors). Under*

www.juliusruechel.com

these circumstances, second generation vaccines with spike protein formulations lacking structurally-conserved ADE-related epitopes should be considered."

In other words, your previous vaccination protects you only until new variants arise, then the training that your previous vaccination gave your immune system becomes a liability as your immune system switches from protecting you to increasing your risk from the disease. Your only way to protect yourself is to dutifully get your next "updated" booster shot to protect you for next few short months. You become a permanent drug dependent vaccine customer. And you better hope next year's formulation doesn't get it wrong. And you better hope that updates can keep you safe indefinitely because there's also the risk that updates will get less effective as the bad training from previous boosters begins to add up.

It puts a whole new spin on "trust the scientists." Your life will literally be at their mercy.

I bet the pharmaceutical industry will be smiling at all those drug-dependent ~~chickens~~ loyal customers though — talk about having a captive audience! And what a sweet deal - vaccine makers have been granted an exemption from liability and, if it goes wrong, they are the go-to guy to solve it... with more boosters.

And with every booster, you'll get to play Russian Roulette all over again with side effects: death, autoimmune diseases, reactivation of dormant viruses, neurological damage, blood clotting, and more. figure 72 shows where the reported side effects on the US VAERS system stand at the time of writing (August 28th, 2021). Make sure you compare these numbers with those shown in figure 43, from only 3 months earlier.

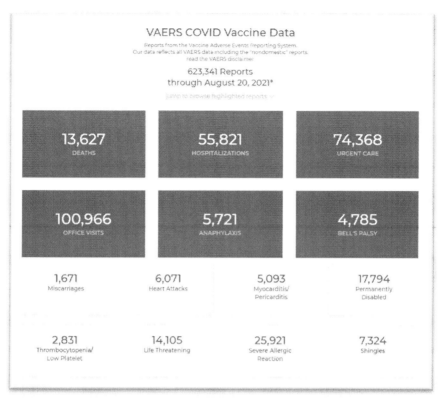

Figure 72: (OpenVaers Search, August 28th, 2021). Compare these numbers with those shown in figure 43, only 3 months earlier.

Leaky vaccines are playing with fire. All vaccine makers and public health authorities were aware of the potential for ADE with the development of a coronavirus vaccine. Yet they pushed for mass vaccination, from day one, without completing the long-term trials that are meant to rule out this kind of risk. They knowingly gambled with your future in their eagerness to get you onto your regimen of never-ending boosters and vaccine passports. Why not, if more boosters are the solution if something going wrong. They can always blame it on the "variants". The media won't challenge them - not with billions of vaccine advertising dollars floating around.

37 — Anti-Virus Security Updates: Cross-Reactive Immunity Through Repeated Exposure

And now we come to the second way in which our immune systems benefit from the rapid evolution of RNA respiratory viruses and to the sinister way in which public health policy is interfering with that system.

The once deadly 1918 Spanish Flu is still with us today; now it is part of the smorgasbord of viruses that cause colds and flus every winter precisely because subsequent variants evolved to be less deadly. As unpleasant as flu season is, for most of us it is not lethal unless we have weak or compromised immune systems. But each subsequent exposure teaches our immune system how to keep up with its gradual evolution over time.

In other words, each year's fresh exposure to the latest strain of cold or flu virus functions as a sort of antivirus security update to partially prepare you for the next one. Fading immunity and changing mutations means you'll never be 100% immune to the next one, but as long as updates are frequent enough, you'll also never have 0% immunity. There will always be enough carry-over to protect you from the most serious outcomes unless you are unfortunate enough to have a weak immune system. That is why it is called *cross-reactive immunity*.

A broad smorgasbord of viruses cruising around during cold and flu season makes it less likely that we will die or get seriously ill when exposed to some new "variant" from London, India, or Brazil, or if we are exposed to a new "cousin", like COVID, which crawls out of some bat cave or wet market or escapes from some lab in Wuhan.

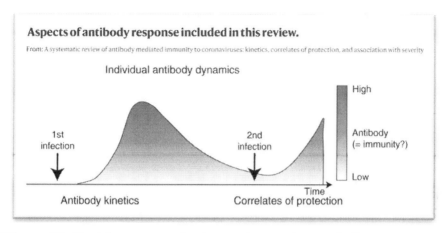

Figure 73: Partial cross-reactive immunity requires periodic re-exposure. (Modified from Huang et al., 2020).

But when we think about it for a moment, what was once dangerous when it was new soon becomes our most important ally for the future to protect us from the next dangerous new thing. As long as we are re-exposed frequently, before immunity fades to zero, cross-reactive immunity is the only realistic evolutionary strategy that humans have to protect us from the next viral variant or viral cousin of these fast-mutating respiratory viruses.

With sufficient leftover cross-reactive immunity from your last exposure, exposure to the latest variant of a virus may simply result in your immune system getting updated without you even noticing a single thing. That's what it means to get an "asymptomatic" infection. Before we started tormenting the healthy with never-ending PCR tests to make us aware of all these "asymptomatic infections", we were constantly getting lots of these "antivirus security updates" each time we encountered one of the more than 200 respiratory viruses circulating among us, often without even noticing the "infection".

Many of these encounters are asymptomatic because our immune systems are able to neutralize them without even ruffling enough layers of our defenses to trigger any symptoms. Almost everyone gets a few immune system updates to the viruses that cause common colds, every single year, yet only a small percentage will ever get very sick. The rest may barely get a runny nose, or no symptoms at all.

Mass PCR testing during COVID created a massive freak-out over every single asymptomatic COVID update when we should have only been focused on those people who come down with severe symptomatic disease. There was never any justifiable reason to roll out PCR tests to asymptomatic citizens other than to heighten fear in the population in order to make them receptive to mass vaccination.

So, in a sense, the 201 respiratory viruses that cause our colds and flus are not just an inconvenience, they are nature's solution to software updates — even though they are dangerous to those with weak immune systems, for the rest of us our immune systems *depend* on them to give us partial protection against new strains that emerge through mutation or when new strains jump across species boundaries. Getting rid of those already circulating in society would make us *more* vulnerable to new variants that emerge. Adding another 200 will make us even safer once we get our first contact behind us.

Eradicating a relatively benign respiratory virus is therefore *not* a desirable goal. But making it fade into the background is a desirable public health goal so that what was once dangerous can now keep protecting us against the next one through cross-reactive immunity. Focused protection for the vulnerable, not lockdowns, was always the only realistic public health response to this respiratory virus, unless someone wanted to seize the opportunity as a way to rope the public into mass vaccinations.

Nature evolved this fascinating strategy of self-updating immunological countermeasures by continually testing us with mild versions of previous closely related respiratory viruses. Our immune system is therefore somewhat similar to an Olympic weightlifter whose muscles not only stay strong but get even stronger by routinely putting his muscles under a little bit of stress. Our immune system functions the same way — it must be continually stress-tested with mild challenges by these fast-mutating viruses in order to develop the robust arsenal of defenses to keep us safe. It is a concept called *anti-fragility,* which was described in detail by Nassim Taleb in his ground-breaking book, *Antifragile: Things That Gain from Disorder.* Once you understand this concept, your fear of "variants" will rapidly dissolve.

The eradication of these fast-mutating respiratory viruses is therefore not just unachievable, it would actually be dangerous if we succeeded because it would eliminate the security updates that we need in order to protect us against new variants that crawl out of bat caves or jump species boundaries. This year's runny nose is your protection against COVID-23. Your cross-reactive immunity to last year's annoying flu might just save your life if something truly dangerous arrives, as long as it is at least somewhat related to what your immune system has seen before. COVID could easily have turned out to be as dangerous to us as the Spanish Flu if it hadn't been for the saving grace of cross-reactive immunity gained from exposure to other coronaviruses. As I've mentioned previously (Majdoubi et al., 2021), up to 90-99% of us already had some level of protection to COVID thanks to partial cross-reactive immunity gained from exposure to other coronaviruses. The high percentage of infections that turn out to be asymptomatic bears that out.

Someone needs to remind Bill Gates, his fawning public health bootlickers, and the pharmaceutical companies that whisper sweet-nothings in his ear that in the natural world of respiratory viruses, most of us don't need a regimen of never-ending booster shots to keep us safe from COVID variants — we already have a perfectly functioning system to keep bringing us new updates. Respiratory viruses are a completely different beast than smallpox, polio, or measles; and pretending otherwise is not just silly, it's criminal because anyone with a background in immunology knows better. But it's a fantastic and very profitably way to scare a wide-eyed population into accepting never-ending booster shots as a replacement for the natural antivirus updates that we normally get from hugs and handshakes. Protect the vulnerable. Stop preying on the rest of us.

38 — The Not-So-Novel Novel Virus: The *Diamond Princess* Cruise Ship Outbreak Proved We Have Cross-Reactive Immunity

A truly *novel* virus affects everyone because no-one has pre-existing cross-reactive partial immunity to it. That's why the diseases that accompanied Christopher Columbus to the Americas killed up to 95% of North and South America's indigenous populations. To them, these diseases were novel because they had no previous exposure to them and therefore lacked the antivirus security updates acquired through pre-existing infections. They would have benefited greatly from access to a vaccine prior to first contact.

Thankfully, COVID-19 was *not* that kind of virus. Yet the media and public health officials shamelessly provoked fear that it was by using the scientifically accurate term *novel* to describe it, knowing full well that all scientists would understand this to mean a newly emergent strain while the general public would jump to the conclusion that this was an entirely new virus (also called a *novel* virus by scientists), like when tuberculosis or influenza accompanied Columbus to the Americas. This was a grotesque example of public health officials misusing scientific terminology, knowing full well that the public would misunderstand the term *novel* according to how we use the word in everyday language and not according to how the scientific community uses it.

That little game successfully sparked a wave of fear that is so strong that, not only is everyone desperate for a leaky jab to lead them to safety, but they are so scared that they won't rest until all their friends, neighbors, and family members get one too even if it requires extreme levels of coercion to get the job done. Canada has even recently gone as far as making vaccination *mandatory* for all federal employees, employees of Crown Corporations, employees of federally regulated companies (i.e. utilities) and for all travelers on commercial airlines and trains (CBC, August 13th, 2021)!

Despite the scary numbers put out by the Chinese government in the early days of the pandemic, the outbreak on the *Diamond Princess* cruise ship served as an inadvertent petri-dish to study the COVID virus. Thanks to that example, by the end of February 2020 we knew that COVID was not some monster virus like the 1918 Spanish Flu but was simply another coronavirus strain that was closely related to previous coronaviruses and that most of us already carried some level of cross-reactive immunity to protect us.

How do we know that? The virus circulated freely onboard the ship, yet age corrected lethality remained between 0.025% and 0.625% (STAT News, March 17, 2020) (that's on the order of a bad flu season and nothing at all like the fatality rate of the 1918 Spanish Flu, which was between 2% and 10%). Only 26% of the passengers tested positive for the virus (Plucinski et al., May 18, 2021) and of those that tested positive 48% remained *completely symptom free* despite the advanced age of most of these passengers (National Institute of Infectious Diseases, Japan, February 19, 2020)!

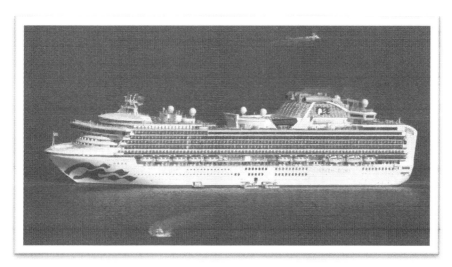

Figure 74: *Diamond Princess* Cruise Ship (image by Alpsdake, CC BY-SA 4.0.)

The *Diamond Princess* didn't turn into the floating morgue of bygone eras when ships carrying a disease were forced into quarantine. That should have been the first clue that this virus was anything but novel in the colloquial understanding of the term. Like most cold and flu viruses, only those with weak immune systems were in danger while everyone else got off with little or no symptoms. That is simply *not* how a truly novel virus behaves when it encounters a population without any pre-existing cross-reactive immunity. The only plausible explanation for that lack of deadliness (deadly for some, annoying for some, and asymptomatic for most others) is that most people already have sufficient pre-existing cross-reactive immunity from exposure to other coronaviruses.

Research subsequently confirmed what the *Diamond Princess* outbreak revealed. Cross-reactive immunity. As I mentioned before, studies have demonstrated that up to 90 - 99% of us already have some residual level of partial protection to COVID (Majdoubi et al., 2021). And we also subsequently found out that most people who were exposed to the deadly SARS virus in 2003 have sufficient residual cross-reactive immunity that they have little to fear from

COVID (Beretta et al., 2020). COVID was never a mortal threat to most of us.

The important thing to remember is that the *Diamond Princess* data was already publicly available since the end of February of 2020. *Operation Warp Speed*, the vaccine development initiative approved by President Trump (Wikipedia, n.d.), was nevertheless announced on April 29th, 2020. Thus, our health authorities knowingly and opportunistically recommended lockdowns and promoted vaccines as an exit strategy *after* it was already clear that the majority of us had some kind of protection through cross-reactive immunity. The *Diamond Princess* example provided the unequivocal proof that the only people who might benefit from a vaccine, even if it worked as advertised, were the small number of extremely vulnerable members of society with weak immune systems. Likewise, lockdowns should have been recommended *only* for nursing home residents (on a strictly *voluntary* basis to protect their human rights) while the pandemic surged through the rest of us.

The only plausible explanation for why our international health authorities ignored the example of the *Diamond Princess* is if they wanted to stoke fear among the public and if they wanted to bamboozle credible politicians in order to opportunistically achieve some other public health agenda. They pushed vaccination on everyone knowing full well that most people don't need it and that protection would fade quickly even if the vaccines had been 100% effective, which they also knew was not going to be the case. And yet they continue to push these vaccines using the same deceitful tactics even today. Water does not run uphill.

> *"We know they are lying,*
> *they know they are lying,*
> *they know we know they are lying,*
> *we know they know we know they are lying,*
> *but they are still lying."*
> — Attributed to Aleksandr Isayevich Solzhenitsyn

39 — Mother Knows Best: Vitamin D, Playing in Puddles, and Sweaters

Just like during other cold and flu seasons, the vulnerable to COVID are overwhelmingly those with compromised immune systems: those whose immune systems are shutting down as they approach death from old age and those whose immune systems are compromised due to severe pre-existing conditions that reduce immune function.

For everyone else with a strong immune system and with cross-reactive immunity, we have little to fear from the virus and its never-ending stream of mutations *unless our immune systems are temporarily suppressed through illness, environmental conditions, or nutritional deficiencies.*

Your mother's warnings about putting on a sweater, hat, and dry socks, tucking in your shirt to cover your kidneys, and not playing in puddles were not about *preventing* infection by a cold or flu, it was about preventing *symptomatic* infection. Research has demonstrated that getting chilled can temporarily suppress your immune system (Harvard Medical School, January 1, 2010). Thus, getting chilled increases the chance that an infection leads to symptomatic disease rather than merely updating your immune system through an asymptomatic infection. Your sweater won't prevent you from catching an infection. But it might prevent that infection from becoming a symptomatic disease. It could be the difference between experiencing nothing and ending up in bed with a fever.

In the same way, topping up on vitamin C and D, eating properly, getting enough rest, getting hugs from loved ones, adopting a positive attitude in life, and smiling when you see a rainbow are all strategies that help keep your immune system strong. They don't prevent infection, but they might reduce your risk of a bad outcome.

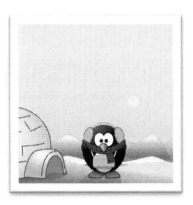

Ask the staff in a nursing home what happens to their patients when any of these important ingredients is missing — vitamin and nutrient deficiencies, poor sleep, loneliness, and depression lay out the welcome mat for the Grim Reaper. A temporarily suppressed immune system cannot mount an adequate immune response even when we do have cross-reactive immunity.

Our public health authorities also all know this. This is not a mystery. Yet, instead of promoting these strategies as ways in which people could reduce their risk to severe outcomes, they have systematically downplayed, ignored, or labeled these strategies as "fake news" (Canadian Health Minister Patty Hajdu, YouTube, April 23rd, 2021). Maximize the risk of death. Then promote the vaccine as the exclusive path to safety. Criminal.

You cannot control other people forever to avoid getting exposed to a respiratory virus. COVID Zero is an authoritarian fantasy. But you can control your food, your sleep, and your attitude so that your immune system can mount the strongest attack it can muster. The odds are that you already have all the cross-reactive immunity you need to survive this virus without a hitch. Look inwards to find freedom from fear. Take good care of yourself. Go play in the sun with your friends. And listen to your mother —tuck in your shirt!

40 — The Paradox: Why COVID-Zero Makes People More Vulnerable to Other Viruses

As is so often the case when politicians try to run our lives for us, the government response to COVID is not just wrong, it is actually making us more vulnerable, both to COVID *and to other respiratory viruses.* Depriving nursing home patients of their loved ones, locking them in isolation, locking people in their homes, shutting down gyms, driving us into depression, and paralyzing us with fear and uncertainty ensures that our immune systems will be working at suboptimal levels. Broken marriages, children deprived of social contacts, insomnia, the remarkable surge in obesity that occurred during COVID, and so many other consequences of these ill begotten strategies all have a toll on our ability to mount a strong immune response when we are inevitably exposed to any respiratory viruses.

Equally devasting is that, by disrupting our normal social contacts, we have reduced how much training our immune system is getting through repeated exposure to other respiratory viruses. A computer that stops getting security updates becomes increasingly vulnerable to future versions of viruses. The same goes for our immune system. COVID is not the only risk. Remember, there are more than 200 other respiratory viruses that are also circulating. They may not be getting much attention and may be temporarily starved for hosts while we are cooped up at home, but they haven't gone away. They are waiting.

And when they find us, they find hosts whose antivirus security updates are out of date.

In other words, by breaking our ability to socialize with our peers, what was once relatively harmless is becoming more dangerous to us because our immune systems are out of practice. This isn't some theoretical risk. We're already beginning to see the fallout from that lack of updates, with deadly consequences.

For example, New Zealand was praised internationally for adopting a COVID-Zero policy and for the low COVID cases that resulted. But the lockdowns, social distancing measures, and border closures also had another effect — there was a 99.9% reduction in flu cases and a 98% reduction in cases of the RSV virus (The Guardian, July 8, 2021). Sounds good, right? Not so fast...

Systems that depend on constant challenges to become antifragile will become fragile if those challenges stop happening. A tree that grows up sheltered from the wind will break when it is exposed to the storm.

Now New Zealand's myopic focus on COVID as the one and only risk is coming home to roost. Its hospitals are overflowing with children. But they're not being hospitalized by COVID. They are falling ill with RSV virus because of the "immunity debt" that built up from not being continually exposed to all the respiratory viruses that make up normal life (The Guardian, July 8, 2021). These children are, quite literally, the next wave of victims of COVID-Zero. Being cut off from normal life has left them fragile. Instead of praise, it now is becoming apparent that New Zealand's authoritarian strongwoman, Jacinda Ardern, and her public health advisors ought to be standing trial for gross negligence for ignoring the long-established research about how our immune systems *depend* on continual exposure to respiratory viruses in order to stay healthy.

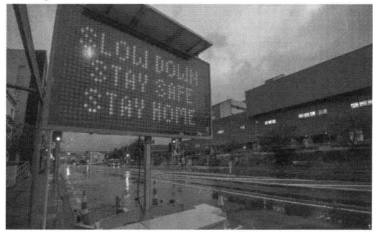

New Zealand children falling ill in high numbers due to Covid 'immunity debt'

Doctors say children haven't been exposed to range of bugs due to lockdowns, distancing and sanitiser and their immune systems are suffering

▲ The Wellington hospital in New Zealand. The city has 46 children hospitalised with respiratory illnesses. Photograph: Dave Lintott/REX/Shutterstock

New Zealand hospitals are experiencing the payoff of "immunity debt" created by Covid-19 lockdowns, with wards flooded by babies with a potentially-deadly respiratory virus, doctors have warned.

Figure 75: (The Guardian, July 8th, 2021).

As long as our social contacts are restricted, we are all becoming increasing vulnerable to all these other respiratory viruses because of the "immunity debt" that has built up during lockdowns and social distancing rules. It turns out that handshakes and hugs are not just good for the soul. Our public health officials have blood on their hands for denying us our normal lives.

This heightened risk to other viruses isn't an unexpected outcome; there were plenty of doctors who warned about precisely this risk as lockdowns were being imposed. For example, Dr. Dan Erickson and Dr Artin Massihi warned about this phenomenon back in May of 2020 (Odysee, May 15th, 2020). YouTube censored their video. Yet they were citing long-established science that was uncontested until society collectively lost its mind in 2020.

41 — Immunity as a Service: A Subscription-Based Business Model for the Pharmaceutical Industry

As you can see from everything I have laid out in this essay, this misbegotten vaccine-enabled fever dream was never a realistic solution to stop COVID. At best, if the vaccines worked as advertised, all they could ever have been was one tool among many to provide the vulnerable with focused protection while the rest of us went about our normal lives, largely unaffected by our periodic antivirus security updates through exposure to the natural virus.

COVID-Zero in all its variations was a fantasy.

But it was not an accidental fantasy.

Water does not run uphill.

Every single public health official in the world has the education to know that what they have been promoting, from day one, is gibberish. What I have laid out in this essay is pretty basic virology and immunology knowledge. Which raises a rather alarming question: how can any virologist, immunologist, vaccine maker, or public health official knowingly promote this lie?

Why is there such a blind obsession with getting us all to take a vaccine that most people do not need and that can never provide long-lasting herd immunity?

It's no mystery why pea-brained politicians might fall for this fantasy; they are only as good as the advisors they listen to. And politicians are shameless opportunists, so it is not surprising that they are now exploiting the situation to increase their powers and to harness this emerging command-and-control economy in pursuit of their own ideological goals — redistribution, carbon net zero, social credit score systems, you name it. In this Orwellian world, if you have a podium and a utopian dream, the world is your oyster, at least as long as the band keeps playing and the pitchforks can be kept off the streets.

"You never let a serious crisis go to waste. And what I mean by that it's an opportunity to do things you think you could not do before." — Rahm Emanuel

"I really believe COVID has created a window of political opportunity..." — Chrystia Freeland, Deputy Prime Minister of Canada

But our public health officials and international health organizations are trained to know better. Yet they nevertheless set this nightmare in motion in violation of all their own long-established pandemic planning guidelines. They *know* eradication is impossible. They *know* most of us already have cross-reactive immunity. They *know* most of us are healthy enough so that our immune systems will protect us against severe outcomes from this virus. They *know* about the negative consequences imposed on our immune systems when we are prevented from living normal lives. They *know* they are increasing our risk to other viruses by preventing us from socializing. It's their job to know. And, as I have demonstrated, they have known since day one.

But what if a shameless pharmaceutical industry could manipulate public health policies by capturing politicians, policymakers, and public health agencies through generous donations? What if the boundaries between public health agencies, international public health organizations, and pharmaceutical companies have become blurred to such a degree that each benefits from reinforcing one another's best interests? What if they have all come to believe that vaccines against respiratory viruses are the holy grail of public health (and of generous funding), even if they have to play fast and loose with the truth to get humanity to accept them and even if they have to do a little evil to achieve some imagined future "greater good"?

What if the revolving door between pharmaceutical companies, public health, and international health organizations has created a kind of blind groupthink within this holy trinity? What if anyone caught up in that system is forced to bite their tongue because to speak out is a deathblow to their career? What if many of those caught up in the system *genuinely* believe the lies, despite a lifetime of training that should tell them otherwise? The powerful effect of groupthink, demonstrated by the *Ash Conformity Experiments* (YouTube, February 20, 2012), can make people blind to what is staring them in the face. Even the medieval kings knew they needed a court jester to prevent the king from growing a big head. But what if, in the hallowed halls of this holy trinity, all the court jesters have long since been purged or cowed into silence?

"It's dangerous to be right when the government is wrong." — Voltaire

A quote that best sums up the thinking inside many of our public health institutions comes from Peter Daszak, head of EcoHealth Alliance, a non-profit non-governmental organization that works closely with public health agencies like the National Institutes of Health (NIH) and intergovernmental organizations like the WHO (The National Academies of Sciences, Engineering, Medicine. February 12, 2016):

"Daszak reiterated that, until an infectious disease crisis is very real, present, and at an emergency threshold, it is often largely ignored. **To sustain funding base beyond the crisis, he said, we need to increase public understanding of the need for MCMs** [*medical counter measures*] **such as a pan-influenza or pan-coronavirus vaccine. A key driver is the media, and the economics follow the hype. We need to use that hype to our advantage to get to the real issues. Investors will respond if they see profit at the end of process**, *Daszak stated." [Emphasis mine]*

In the presence of so much conflict of interest, in the absence of the checks and balances provided by individual rights, in the censorious atmosphere of cancel culture that has infected all our public institutions, and with so many institutional donors (private and governmental alike) being enamored with social-engineering projects and blinded by their own arrogance, it would perhaps be more surprising if this vaccine-fueled hysteria *hadn't* happened.

In view of the circumstances, what happened almost seems inevitable. To the eyes of profit-hungry pharmaceuticals and funding-hungry national and international public health institutions, this virus must look like manna from heaven. They must feel like a fox that has been invited into the henhouse by ripe chickens that are begging to be plucked.

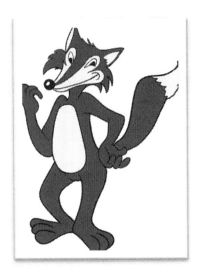

History never repeats itself, but it does often rhyme. What has emerged during COVID is simply a bigger, better, bolder replay of what happened during the 2009 swine flu hysteria. I'd like to share a few quotes with you - and keep in mind that these are about the 2009 Swine Flu scandal, not COVID:

From a 2010 article entitled: *European Parliament to Investigate WHO and "Pandemic" Scandal* (healthcare-in-europe.com, January 26, 2010) [Emphasis mine]:

> *"In his official statement to the Committee, Wodarg* **criticized the influence of the pharma industry on scientists and officials of [the] WHO**, *stating that it has led to the situation where* **"unnecessarily millions of healthy people are exposed to the risk of poorly tested vaccines,"** *and that, for a flu strain that is "vastly less harmful" than all previous flu epidemics."*

> *"For the first time, the* **WHO criteria for a pandemic was changed in April 2009** *as the first Mexico cases were reported, to make not the actual risk of a disease but the number of cases of the disease [the] basis to declare "Pandemic."* **By classifying the swine flu as [a] pandemic, nations were compelled to implement pandemic plans and also t[o] purchase swine flu vaccines."**

And here are a series of even more revealing quotes from a 2010 report published by *Der Spiegel* called: *Reconstruction of a Mass Hysteria — The Swine Flu Panic of 2009* (Spiegel International, 2010):

"Researchers in more than 130 laboratories in 102 countries are constantly on the lookout for new flu pathogens. Entire careers and institutions, and a lot of money, depend on the outcomes of their work. **"Sometimes you get the feeling that there is a whole industry almost waiting for a pandemic to occur,"** *says flu expert Tom Jefferson, from an international health nonprofit called the Cochrane Collaboration. "And all it took was one of these influenza viruses to mutate to start the machine grinding."*

"Does this mean that a very mild course of the pandemic was not even considered from the start? At any rate, **efforts to downplay the risks were unwelcome, and the WHO made it clear that it preferred to base its decisions on a worst-case scenario.** *"We wanted to overestimate rather than underestimate the situation," says Fukuda [Keiji Fukuda was the Assistant Director-General for Health, Security and Environment for the WHO at that time]."*

"The media also did its part in stoking fears. *SPIEGEL, for example, had reported at length on the avian flu. Now it devoted a cover story to the new "global virus," a story filled with concerns that the swine flu pathogen could mutate into a horrific virus."*

"The pharmaceutical industry was particularly adept at keeping this vision alive."

"We expected a real pandemic, and we thought that it had to happen. **There was no one who suggested re-thinking our approach."**

"the vast majority of experts on epidemics automatically associate the term "pandemic" with truly aggressive viruses. On the WHO Web site, the

www.juliusruechel.com

answer to the question "*What is a pandemic?*" included mention of "*an enormous number of deaths and cases of the disease*" -- until May 4, 2009. That was when a CNN reporter pointed out the discrepancy between this description and the generally mild course of the swine flu. **The language was promptly removed**."

"'*Sometimes some of us think that WHO stands for World Hysteria Organization*,' says Richard Schabas, the former chief medical officer for Canada's Ontario Province."

"*A party with strong connections in Geneva had a strong interest in phase 6 being declared as quickly as possible: the pharmaceutical industry.*"

"*Meanwhile, a debate had erupted over whether Germany had chosen the wrong vaccine, Pandemrix [it was later found to have caused narcolepsy in some patients, which is an autoimmune disease]. It contained a new type of agent designed to boost its effectiveness, known as an adjuvant, **which had never undergone large-scale human trials** in connection with the swine flu antigen. Were millions of people about to receive a vaccine that had hardly been tested?*"

"But **the contracts for Pandemrix had been signed in 2007, and they came into effect automatically when the WHO decided to declare phase 6**."

"**The ministers felt pressured from all sides**. On the one hand, **the media were stoking fears of the virus**. The German tabloid newspaper Bild, in particular, was printing new tales of horror almost daily. On the other hand, **the pharmaceutical companies were upping the pressure and constantly setting new ultimatums**."

"*Oct. 9, 2009: Wolf-Dieter Ludwig, an oncologist and chairman of the Drug Commission of the German Medical Association, says:* '*The* **health authorities have fallen for a campaign by the** *pharmaceutical companies, which were plainly using a supposed threat to make money."'*

*"Oct. 21, 2009: A BILD newspaper headline, printed in toxic yellow, warns: "Swine Flu Professor Fears 35,000 Dead in Germany !" The professor's name is Adolf Windorfer, and when pressed, **he admits that he has received payments from the industry**, including GSK and Novartis. **Next to the BILD headline is an ad for the German Association of Pharmaceutical Companies**."*

*"According to Wodarg, **the WHO's classification of the swine flu as a pandemic have earned the pharmaceutical companies $18 billion in additional revenues.** Annual sales of Tamiflu alone have jumped 435 percent, to €2.2 billion."*

Rinse and repeat in 2020-2021.

What if, upon recognizing the emergence of a new pandemic, those in the know opportunistically made vaccines the endgame? What if all the vaccine injuries recorded on VAERS and all the risks they are taking with our lives are simply collateral damage - a calculated investment risk - in order to turn their dream of subscription-based "immunity as a service" into reality.

In the words of Bill Gates, *"we kind of caught mRNA halfway to prime time."* (YouTube, March 10, 2021). Maybe we should believe him — and gape in awe at the recklessness and contempt they have shown for their fellow citizens in order to capitalize on this "window of opportunity". Carpe diem (seize the day). Don't sweat the small stuff. Keep your eye on the ball... and on the year-end bonuses.

What if COVID-Zero, in all its variations, was merely a strategy to herd us together so we obediently line up for an endless string of booster shots as a trade-off for access to our lives?

In other words, what if someone could bamboozle our leaders into believing that the only way back to a normal life is for vaccines to *replace* the role that hugs and handshakes used to play in order to update us with the latest antivirus security updates?

What if, by depriving us of normal life, those who stand to gain from vaccines can forever cement themselves at the center of society by providing an artificial replacement for what our immune systems used to do to protect us against common respiratory viruses back when we were still allowed to live normal lives?

The headlines tell the story:

"Pfizer CEO says third Covid vaccine dose likely needed within 12 months." (CNBC, April 15th, 2021)

"Variants could be named after star constellations when Greek alphabet runs out, says WHO Covid chief." (The Telegraph, August 7th, 2021)

"Fauci warns Americans may face having booster shots indefinitely" (Daily Mail, August 13th, 2021) and (Dr. Fauci in his own words on YouTube on August 12th, 2021)

"Biden OKs booster shots 5 months after 2nd dose" (Boston Globe, August 27th, 2021)

What if the fast mutation of RNA viruses ensures that no vaccine will ever be fully effective at providing lasting immunity, thus creating the illusion that we are permanently in need of vaccine boosters as long as the public can be kept in fear?

What if politicians could be convinced to make vaccination mandatory in order to prevent potential customers from opting out?

What if, by relying on lockdowns during the winter season, our vulnerability to other viruses increased, which could then be used to rationalize expanding the jab, via mission creep, to simultaneously vaccinate us against RSV, influenza, other coronaviruses, the common cold, and so on, despite knowing full well that the protection that these vaccines offer against respiratory viruses is only temporary?

Moderna Announces Positive Pre-Clinical Data for Single Shot Combining COVID, RSV & Flu Vaccines (CBS New York, September 10th, 2021)

And what other social engineering goals can be rolled into your annual booster shot in the future once you are permanently bound to these annual jabs and vaccine passports? In an atmosphere of hysteria, it's a system ripe for abuse by opportunists, ideologues, power hungry totalitarians, and Malthusian social engineers. The snowball doesn't have to grow by design. Mission creep happens all on its own once Pandora's Box is opened to coerced vaccinations and conditional rights. The road to Hell is frequently paved by good intentions... and hysteria.

So, what if COVID-Zero and the vaccine exit strategy is merely the global state-sanctioned equivalent of a drug dealer creating dependency among its customers to keep pushing more drugs?

What if it all started as a way of convincing society of the need for subscription-based "immunity as a service"? The subscription-based business model (or some version of it) is all the rage these days in the corporate world to create loyal captive audiences that generate reliable money streams, forever. Subscriptions are not just for your cable TV and gym membership anymore. Everything has been redesignated as a "consumable".

- Netflix did it with movies.

- Spotify did it with music.

- Microsoft did it with its Office suite.

- Adobe did it with its Photoshop editing suite.

- The smartphone industry did it with phones that need to be replaced every 3 to 5 years.

- The gaming industry did it with video games.

- Amazon is doing it with books (i.e. Kindle Unlimited).

- The food industry is doing it with meal delivery services (i.e. Hello Fresh).

- Uber is doing it with subscription-based ride sharing.

- Coursera is doing it with online education.

- Duolingo and Rosetta Stone are doing it with language learning.

- Zoom is doing it with online meetings.

- Monsanto and its peers did it to farmers with patented seed technology, which cannot legally be replanted, and is lobbying to try to legalize the use of terminator seed technology (GMO seeds that are sterile in the second generation to prevent replanting).

- The healthcare industry is doing it with concierge medical services (Ntc Texas, 2019), fitness tracking apps (Fitbit), sleep-tracking apps, and meditation apps.

- The investment industry is doing it with farmland, with investors owning the land and leasing it back to farmers in a kind of modern revival of the sharecropping system. (Bill Gates is the largest farmland owner in the USA (Business Insider, May 4, 2021) - are you surprised?)

- Blackrock and other investment firms are currently trying to do it with single family homes to create a permanent class of renters (Twitter, June 8, 2021).

- And public health authorities and vaccine makers have been trying to do it with flu vaccines for years, but we've been stubbornly uncooperative. Not anymore.

Remember when the World Economic Forum predicted in 2016 that by 2030 all products would become services? (World Economic Forum, November 12, 2016) And remember their infamous video in which they predicted that "You will own nothing. And you will be happy."? Well, the future is here. This is what it looks like. The subscription-based economy. And apparently it now also includes your immune system in a trade-off for access to your life.

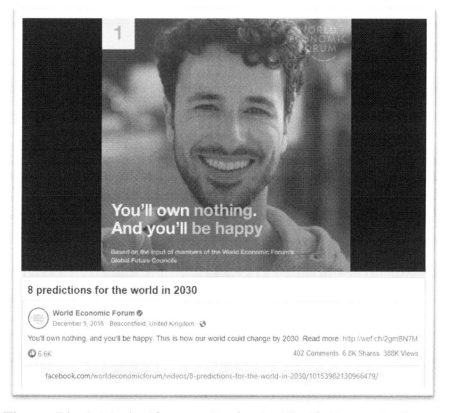

Figure 76: Original video on Facebook (World Economic Forum, December 9, 2016).

Let's revisit the Peter Daszak quote from earlier. A second read allows the message to really hit home:

"Daszak reiterated that, until an infectious disease crisis is very real, present, and at an emergency threshold, it is often largely ignored. **To sustain the funding base beyond the crisis, he said, we need to increase public understanding of the need for MCMs** *[medical counter measures]* **such as a pan-influenza or a pan-coronavirus vaccine. A key driver is the media, and the economics follow the hype. We need to use that hype to our advantage to get to the real issues. Investors will respond if they see profit at the end of process**, *Daszak stated."*

Isn't it ironic that he didn't even care which vaccine was pushed? Influenza or coronavirus, it made no difference. It was always about funding. It was always about the money. It always was. It always is.

The holy trinity of pharmaceutical companies, public health, and international health organizations, all egging each other on in their hunger for a reliable flow of cash: shareholder profits, larger budgets, and governmental donations. Their interests are perfectly aligned and the lines between them are blurred to such a degree that each benefits from reinforcing one another's best interests.

And why would politicians and media bow to the holy trinity?

Big Pharma spent an average of US$4.7 billion per year between 1999 and 2018 on lobbying and campaign contributions, just in the USA (Wouters, 2020)!

Big Pharma also shells out $US20 billion each year to schmooze doctors and another US$6 billion on drug ads, just in the USA (ARS Technica, January 11, 2019)! So, it's no surprise that legacy media and Big Tech are tripping over themselves not to ruffle the party line — they live and die by the almighty pharmaceutical advertising dollar. Never bite the hand that feeds you.

So, they are all dancing to the same tune while your pocket gets picked and your arm gets pricked, and everyone wins... except you and me. We are the cow that gets milked. We are the serfs that fund their largesse in this neo-feudal society where a few big boys own the assets and everyone else is beholden to those above them in the hierarchy for access to, well, everything — land, resources, rights, individual autonomy, and even immune systems. My body, their choice.

What if, in an atmosphere of runaway hysteria, a police state founded on medical tyranny is creating itself, fueled by a toxic brew of self-serving opportunists who have seized the moment to superimpose their own goals on a fortuitous virus until one day you wake up to find yourself chained and milked, like a cow in a dairy barn, under the absolute custody of a modern-day Louis the Fourteenth and his royal court full of drug pushers, ideologues, and militant devotees? The modern face of feudalism, updated for the 21st century. Neo-feudalism, enforced by a mandatory subscription-based "immunity as a service".

And what if a society that has lost its principles, a society that is eager to hand over individual responsibility to "experts," a society that is held hostage to cancel culture mobs, a society that no longer has transparency into the decisions made by its experts, a society led by a censorious political class full of immoral opportunists, a society that has fallen so in love with big government that red tape and cronyism have completely erased the self-limiting checks and balances of a free and open society, and a society that has elevated "safetyism" to a new sort of religious cult is a society that has no immunity to protect itself from predators who treat us like cattle?

No period in history has ever lacked in snake-oil salesmen, ideologues, and social engineers eager to take society for a ride. Most of the time, they are ignored. So, what if the only real mystery is why society has grown so willing to accept the collar and yoke?

What if all this really is just as simple as that?

42 — The Path Forward: Neutralizing the Threat and Bullet-Proofing Society to Prevent This Ever Happening Again.

Now we know we've been played, how we've been played, and why we've been played. Again. Just like during the 2009 Swine Flu con. Only bigger, bolder, and better. They learned from their mistakes. We didn't.

But now that you see the con, you can't unsee it. And now that you understand the threat and how the game is being played, there is a weight that comes off your shoulders.

When you know there is a threat stalking you but you don't know exactly what it is, every movement in the grass might be a tiger or a snake or a scorpion. It's paralyzing and exhausting to defend yourself against an invisible unknown and they have used that fear masterfully against us to keep us frozen. But once you spot the tiger in the grass, you know where to direct your focus, your feet become unglued, your voice becomes bold, and you regain the clarity of thought to defend yourself.

The con is clear. Now it's time to focus all our might on stopping this runaway train before it takes us over the cliff into a police state of no return. Stand up. Speak out. Refuse to play along. Stopping this requires millions of voices with the courage to say NO — at work, at home, at school, at church, and out on the street.

"Nonviolent direct action seeks to create such a crisis & foster such a tension that a community which has constantly refused to negotiate is forced

to confront the issue. It seeks so to dramatize the issue that it can no longer be ignored." — Martin Luther King Jr.

Compliance is the glue that holds tyranny together. Non-compliance breaks it apart. One person alone cannot stop this. But if millions find the courage to raise their voices and the courage to refuse to participate in the system on these tyrannical medical terms, it will throw the system into such a crisis and create such a tension that the community will be forced to confront the issue. Without enough truckers, no-one eats. Without enough medical staff, hospitals close. Without enough workers, supply chains break. Without enough policemen, oppressive laws cannot be enforced. Without enough garbage collectors, cities grind to a halt. Without enough cashiers, box stores cannot stay open. Without enough administrators, institutions cease to function. Without enough staff, corporations lose profits. Without enough servers, restaurants cannot serve their customers. And without enough customers, businesses are brought to their knees.

Tyranny is not sustainable if the system grinds to a halt. Make it grind by being a thorn in everyone's side until they give us back our freedoms and end this ridiculous charade. They are trying to impose vaccine passports and mandatory vaccinations. But we hold the cards... but only if we are bold enough to stand up even at the risk of finding ourselves standing alone. Courage begets courage. It was Martin Luther King's secret power. It must be ours.

Now that you see the con, you also know the simple recipe to make this virus go away before their reckless policies turn it a monster virus for real. Remember 1918. End the war on the virus. Let the young folks come out of the trenches. Let people go back to their lives. Provide focused protection for the vulnerable. That is how this virus fades into the history books.

It's time to be bold. It's time to call out the fraudsters. And it's time to reclaim the habits, values, and principles that are required to fix our democratic and scientific institutions to prevent this from ever happening again.

Feudalism was one giant stinking cesspool of self-serving corruption. Individual rights, free markets, the democratic process, and limited government were the antidotes that freed humanity from that hierarchical servitude. It seems we have come full circle. The COVID con is a symptom, not the cause, of a broken system.

Modern liberal democracy all around the world was inspired by the system of checks and balances that America's Founding Fathers built to prevent government from being co-opted by the special interests of its leaders, institutions, corporations, and most influential citizens. The ink was barely dry when those principles began to be ignored by those with ever greater enthusiasm for an all-powerful referee to manage even the most intimate details of how everyone lives their lives. After two and a half centuries of effort the admirers of big government have achieved their heart's desire. And what a glorious and rotten cesspool of self-serving corruption it is.

But the principles laid out by America's Founding Fathers remain as true today as the day they were written and are waiting to be rediscovered. If there is one culprit who deserves to shoulder more blame than any other for the fiasco of the last 18 months, it is society itself for allowing itself to fall prey to the siren song of big government, the illusion that there can ever be a benevolent, virtuous, and incorruptible referee. He who creates the red tape, he who has the keys to the treasury, he who wields the power of the tax collector, and he who commands those sent to enforce the laws will always have an entourage of self-serving charlatans, rent seekers, and parasites whispering in his ear wherever he goes. So, keep his powers on a very short leash to keep other people's hands off your money, your property, your freedom, and your body. You don't need better leaders. You need less powerful institutions. That's how you prevent this from ever happening again.

Freedom of speech, individual rights, private property, individual ownership, competition, good faith debate, small government, minimal taxes, limited regulation, and free markets (the opposite of the crony capitalism we suffer under now), these are the checks and balances that bullet-proof a society against the soulless charlatans that fail upwards into positions of power in bloated government institutions and against the parasitic fraudsters that seek to attach themselves to the government's teat.

Yes, we need a Great Reset. Just not the subscription-based version that the World Economic Forum imagined.

"One of the saddest lessons of history is this: If we've been bamboozled long enough, we tend to reject any evidence of the bamboozle. We're no longer interested in finding out the truth. The bamboozle has captured us. It's simply too painful to acknowledge, even to ourselves, that we've been taken. Once you give a charlatan power over you, you almost never get it back." — Carl Sagan, The Demon-Haunted World: Science as a Candle in the Dark

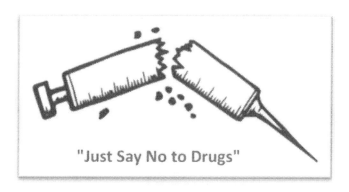

"Just Say No to Drugs"

Acknowledgements

Watching the chaos of the past year and a half leads to the impression that science has died and that democracy has been extinguished. But what makes both work are people, not the institutions that we have built around them. The institutions are rotten to the core and desperately need to be reformed. But the freedom to think and to speak, without reservation, and the no-holds-barred gauntlet of debate, which is essential to the healthy functioning of both science and democracy, are still happening. The human spirit always finds a way to carve out a bubble beyond the reach of chains.

Social media and the internet have emerged as the host for this Wild Wild West of ideas, creating a peer review process so utterly unfiltered that no idea can go unchallenged or become irreversibly corrupted by political or institutional influence. Despite governments' best efforts to censor the conversation and despite Big Tech's best efforts to moderate what can be said out loud, the internet is still a place where known public figures, the leading minds of this age, and the most anonymous of citizens are all put on a level playing field. In this realm, it's the quality of ideas not the credentials of those who utter them which rule the day.

If the Age of Enlightenment found its origins in the rough and tumble of publishing houses and in the networks of curious minds spreading ideas around the globe, then we are witnessing a similar grassroots phenomenon happening today as the human spirit pushes back against the chains imposed from above. This is how the revival of our institutions will begin. And over the past year and a half, I have been privileged to be part of this growing community of independent thinkers. If there is a silver lining to the madness of the past year and a half, it is all the extraordinary people that I have met, both publicly and privately, who are united in their passion for freedom, their strong moral compass, their unrelenting drive to dig into the details, their dedication to treating people as individuals, and their commitment to independent thought.

We have shared ideas, helped each other in our research, and put one another on the hot seat. Many of the people in this community have become genuine friends and it has become a support network unlike any other I have ever been part of. Their ideas, their research, their emails and comments, their willingness to track down information, and their willingness to wrestle with ideas have become invaluable to me. A giant "Thank You" to all of you.

At the risk of leaving out many important voices, there are a number of people and organizations that I would like to thank in particular: @Milhouse_Van_Ho, Trish Wood (trishwoodpodcast.com), Police On Guard For Thee (policeonguard.ca), Len Faul, Russ Cooper, Canadian Citizens for Charter Rights and Freedoms (canadiancitizens.org), Vaccine Choice Canada (vaccinechoicecanada.com), Ted Kuntz, Dr. Peter Breggin (breggin.com), Abir Ballan (@AbirBallan), Kate Wand (veryopinionated.com), Nick Hudson (pandata.org), Kelly Brown (@rubiconcapital_), Donald Welsh (@DonaldWelsh16), Jean Marc Benoit (@JeanmarcBenoit), Julie Ponesse, Marta Gameiro, Voices for Freedom (voicesforfreedom.co.nz), The Briar Patch Observatory (briarpod.net), Will Dove, and Strong and Free Canada (strongandfreecanada.org). And then there are the many many private citizens, online and off, who I shall not name in person to avoid creating a list for the censors, but you know who you are and the immense contributions you have made to my writing. I thank you all for your tireless encouragement, support, and feedback – I am honored to have met all of you! And last but not least, a big "Thank

You" to my wife, Anne, who has cracked the whip, wielded the editor's pencil, and kept me from losing sight of the little things that keep the smiles and the laughter bright even on the darkest of days.

Additional Notes

[1]Calculations for Figure 9, 12, 13, 14, 15, 16, and 17:

Calculations + formulas, based on the original outbreak data set shown in Figure 8:

Setting	outbreaks	cases	deaths	Figure 9: # cases per outbreak	Figure 13 + 14: Deaths per 100 cases	Figure 15: Deaths by Setting (% of total)
Community (cities, towns, reserves, colonies)	229	15,181	141	66	0.928793	1.0
Corrections/shelter/congregate living	796	14,455	226	18	1.563473	1.6
Food/drink/retail	756	3,013	3	4	0.099569	0.0
Hospitals, healthcare	850	11,134	844	13	7.580384	6.1
Industrial (incl. Agriculture)	651	14,903	25	23	0.167751	0.2
LTC & retirement	4,643	67,806	12,541	15	18.495413	90.9
Personal care	61	747	0	12	0.000000	0.0
School & Childcare	1,348	9,016	1	6	0.011091	0.0
Other (gatherings, office work, gyms, etc)	664	6,017	8	9	0.132957	0.1
	10,198	142,272	13,789	=F/E	=G/F*100	=G/G14*100

Figure 16: 2 populations	Figure 17: 2 populations
Deaths in institutions (%)	Deaths in institutions (#)
98.71	13,611
=(G6+G8+G10)/G14*100	=G6+G8+G10
Deaths in the community (%)	Deaths in the community (#)
1.29	178
=(G5+G7+G9+G11+G12+G13)/G14*100	=(G5+G7+G9+G11+G12+G13)

Figure 77: Calculations for Figure 9, 12, 13, 14, 15, 16, and 17. Using data from figure 8.

[2]The world bank estimates that there are 2.52 hospital beds in Canada per 1000 (The World Bank, n.d.), Statistics Canada puts Canada's population at 38 million (Statistics Canada, July 1st, 2020).

[3]Hospital utilization rates in Ontario during COVID (leaked chart from official sources. The authenticity is unconfirmed but is supported by publicly available statements about hospital capacity both before and after the pandemic, as I documented in my article called *Bystander at the Switch: The Moral Case Against Lockdowns*. (www.juliusruechel.com, January 29, 2021):

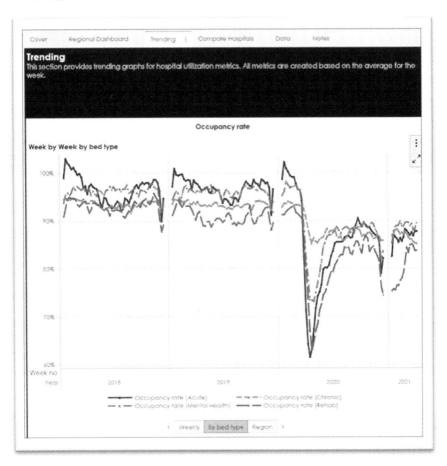

Figure 78: Ontario hospital occupancy rates never rose above 90% throughout the pandemic (@Milhouse_Van_Ho, Twitter, April 15th, 2021).

[4]Ontario's bed capacity is also mirrored by official data from the UK's NHS England, which lends additional weight to its credibility:

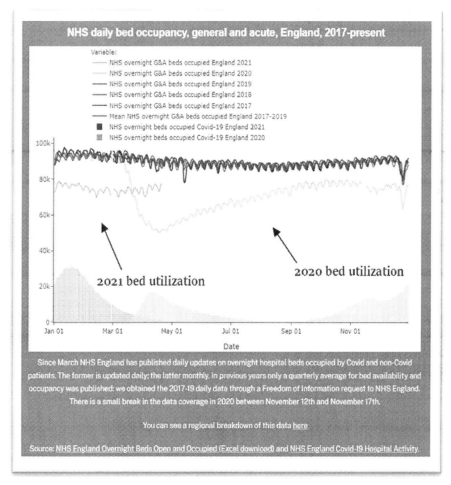

Figure 79: : NHS daily bed occupancy, general and acute, England, 2017-present (Coviddashboard - Data from NHS England, n.d.)

[5]Canada's Age Pyramid:

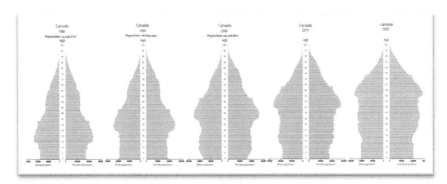

Figure 80: Canada's Age Pyramid, by decade, 1980 to 2020. (Statistics Canada, n.d.)

[6, 7, 8]The Nuremberg Code (British Medical Journal, 1996): (learn more about the Nuremberg Code, its history, and its impact on international law on Wikipedia. (Wikipedia, n.d.):

1. The voluntary consent of the human subject is absolutely essential. This means that the person involved should have legal capacity to give consent; should be so situated as to be able to exercise free power of choice, without the intervention of any element of force, fraud, deceit, duress, overreaching, or other ulterior form of constraint or coercion; and should have sufficient knowledge and comprehension of the elements of the subject matter involved as to enable him to make an understanding and enlightened decision. This latter element requires that before the acceptance of an affirmative decision by the experimental subject there should be made known to him the nature, duration, and purpose of the experiment; the method and means by which it is to be conducted; all inconveniences and hazards reasonably to be expected; and the effects upon his health or person which may possibly come from his participation in the experiment. The duty and responsibility for ascertaining the quality of the consent rests upon each individual who initiates, directs, or engages in the experiment. It is a personal duty and responsibility which may not be delegated to another with impunity.

2. The experiment should be such as to yield fruitful results for the good of society, unprocurable by other methods or means of study, and not random and unnecessary in nature.

3. The experiment should be so designed and based on the results of animal experimentation and a knowledge of the natural history of the disease or other problem under study that the anticipated results justify the performance of the experiment.

4. The experiment should be so conducted as to avoid all unnecessary physical and mental suffering and injury.

5. No experiment should be conducted where there is an a priori reason to believe that death or disabling injury will occur; except, perhaps, in those experiments where the experimental physicians also serve as subjects.

6. The degree of risk to be taken should never exceed that determined by the humanitarian importance of the problem to be solved by the experiment.

7. Proper preparations should be made and adequate facilities provided to protect the experimental subject against even remote possibilities of injury, disability or death.

8. The experiment should be conducted only by scientifically qualified persons. The highest degree of skill and care should be required through all stages of the experiment of those who conduct or engage in the experiment.

9. During the course of the experiment the human subject should be at liberty to bring the experiment to an end if he has reached the physical or mental state where continuation of the experiment seems to him to be impossible.

10. During the course of the experiment the scientist in charge must be prepared to terminate the experiment at any stage, if he has probable cause to believe, in the exercise of the good faith, superior skill and careful judgment required of him, that a continuation of the experiment is likely to result in injury, disability, or death to the experimental subject.

References

Introduction: "Houston, We Have a Problem"

Ioannidis, J. (2020, March 17). A fiasco in the making? As the coronavirus pandemic takes hold, we are making decisions without reliable data. *STAT News*. Retrieved from: https://www.statnews.com/2020/03/17/a-fiasco-in-the-making-as-the-coronavirus-pandemic-takes-hold-we-are-making-decisions-without-reliable-data/

Eschenbach, W. (2020, March 16). Diamond Princess Mysteries. Retrieved from *Wattsupwiththat.com*: https://wattsupwiththat.com/2020/03/16/diamond-princess-mysteries/

Lewis, N. (2020, March 25). COVID-19: Updated data implies that UK modelling hugely overestimates the expected death rates from infection. Retrieved from *JudithCurry.com*: https://judithcurry.com/2020/03/25/covid-19-updated-data-implies-that-uk-modelling-hugely-overestimates-the-expected-death-rates-from-infection/

Bendavid et al. (2020, April 11). COVID-19 Antibody Seroprevalence in Santa Clara County, California. *Medrxiv.org*. Retrieved from https://www.medrxiv.org/content/10.1101/2020.04.14.20062463v1.full.pdf

Ioannidis, J. (2021, March 26). Reconciling estimates of global spread and infection fatality rates of COVID-19: An overview

of systematic evaluations. *European Journal of Clinical Investigation.*
Retrieved from
https://onlinelibrary.wiley.com/doi/10.1111/eci.13554

Humphreys, A. (2020, March 14). What might our lives look like
when Canada is in the full grip of COVID-19? *National Post.*
Retrieved from: https://nationalpost.com/news/may-soon-be-completely-out-of-control-covid-19s-dire-possibilities-could-dramatically-change-canada

Hardingham-Gill, T. (2020, March 11). Naomi Campbell wears
hazmat suit to airport amid coronavirus outbreak. *CNN.*
Retrieved from: https://www.cnn.com/travel/article/naomi-campbell-coronavirus-precaution-outfit/index.html

WHO (2019, November 19). Global Influenza Programme. *Non-pharmaceutical public health measures for mitigating the risk and impact of epidemic and pandemic influenza.* Retrieved from
https://apps.who.int/iris/bitstream/handle/10665/329438/9
789241516839-eng.pdf?ua=1

1 — Prologue:

Carrigg, D. (2021, April 19). Infant dies from COVID-19 at B.C.
Children's Hospital. *Vancouver Sun.* Retrieved from
https://vancouversun.com/news/local-news/infant-dies-from-covid-19-at-b-c-childrens-hospital

Our World Data. (2021, May 7). Daily new confirmed COVID-19
deaths per million people. *Our World Data.* Retrieved from
https://ourworldindata.org/explorers/coronavirus-data-explorer?zoomToSelection=true&time=2020-03-01..latest&pickerSort=desc&pickerMetric=new_deaths_per_m
illion&Metric=Confirmed+deaths&Interval=7-day+rolling+average&Relative+to+Population=true&Align+o
utbreaks=false&country=~CAN

Statistics Canada. (2021, May 20). *Leading causes of death, total
population, by age group.* Retrieved May 20, 2021, from Statistics

Canada: https://web.archive.org/web/20210520053020/https:/www1 50.statcan.gc.ca/t1/tbl1/en/tv.action?pid=1310039401&pick Members%5B0%5D=2.1&pickMembers%5B1%5D=3.1&cub eTimeFrame.startYear=2015&cubeTimeFrame.endYear=2019 &referencePeriods=20150101%2C20190101

Government of Canada. (2021, May 8). *COVID-19 daily epidemiology update*. Retrieved from Coronavirus disease (COVID-10): https://web.archive.org/web/20210509074839if_/https:/healt h-infobase.canada.ca/covid-19/epidemiological-summary-covid-19-cases.html

Provincial Health Services Authority. (n.d.). *BC Children's Hospital - About - Our Unique Role*. Retrieved May 29, 2021, from BC Children's Hospital: http://www.bcchildrens.ca/about/our-unique-role

Weichel, A. (2021, April 19). Toddler becomes youngest person to die of COVID-19 in B.C.. *CTV News*. Retrieved from https://bc.ctvnews.ca/toddler-becomes-youngest-person-to-die-of-covid-19-in-b-c-1.5392989

Statistics Canada. (2021, July 6). Population estimates on July 1st, by age and sex. *Statistics Canada*. Retrieved from https://www150.statcan.gc.ca/t1/tbl1/en/tv.action?pid=1310 039401&pickMembers%5B0%5D=2.1&pickMembers%5B1% 5D=3.1&cubeTimeFrame.startYear=2015&cubeTimeFrame.e ndYear=2019&referencePeriods=20150101%2C20190101

WHO (2019, November 19). Global Influenza Programme. *Non-pharmaceutical public health measures for mitigating the risk and impact of epidemic and pandemic influenza*. Retrieved from https://apps.who.int/iris/bitstream/handle/10665/329438/9 789241516839-eng.pdf?ua=1

2 — A Little Housekeeping: Open Statements

Government of Canada. (2021, February 17). *National case definition: Coronavirus disease (COVID-19).* Retrieved from Government of Canada: https://www.canada.ca/en/public-health/services/diseases/2019-novel-coronavirus-infection/health-professionals/national-case-definition.html

Public Health Agency of Canada. (2021, April 30). *CANADA COVID-19 WEEKLY EPIDEMIOLOGY REPORT 18 APRIL TO 24 APRIL 2021 (WEEK 16).* Retrieved from www.canada.ca: https://web.archive.org/web/20210501003054/https:/www.canada.ca/content/dam/phac-aspc/documents/services/diseases/2019-novel-coronavirus-infection/surv-covid19-weekly-epi-update-20210430-eng.pdf

3 — How Big Are Outbreaks in Different Settings?

Statistics Canada. (2021, July 6). International travelers entering or returning to Canada, by type of transport. *Statistics Canada.* Retrieved from https://www150.statcan.gc.ca/t1/tbl1/en/tv.action?pid=2410004101&pickMembers%5B0%5D=1.1&cubeTimeFrame.startMonth=03&cubeTimeFrame.startYear=2020&cubeTimeFrame.endMonth=02&cubeTimeFrame.endYear=2021&referencePeriods=20200301%2C20210201

Nuttall, J. (2021, May, 7). Governments across Canada withholding COVID-19 data to regulate public reaction to pandemic, says access-to-information advocate. *Toronto Star.* Retrieved from https://www.thestar.com/news/canada/2021/05/07/governments-across-canada-withholding-covid-19-data-to-regulate-public-reaction-to-pandemic-says-access-to-information-advocate.html?utm_source=Twitter&utm_medium=SocialMedia&utm_campaign=National&utm_content=governments-withholding-

data&utm_source=twitter&source=torontostar&utm_medium
=SocialMedia&utm_campaign=&utm_campaign_id=&utm_co
ntent=

7 — Why Are So Few People Dying Outside of Institutions?

Cha, A. E. (2020, August 8). Forty percent of people with coronavirus infections have no symptoms. Might they be the key to ending the pandemic? *Washington Post*. Retrieved from https://www.washingtonpost.com/health/2020/08/08/asymptomatic-coronavirus-covid/

8 — Captive Populations vs The Rest of the Community

Howlett, K. (2021, April 22). Ontario hospitals transfer patients to long-term care to free up beds for COVID patients. *The Globe and Mail*. Retrieved from https://www.theglobeandmail.com/canada/article-ontario-hospitals-transfer-patients-to-long-term-care-to-free-up-beds/

Brown, D. (2020, August 18). Staff living with nursing home residents with COVID-19 reduced deaths, cases: study. *McKnight's Long-term Care News*. Retrieved from https://www.mcknights.com/news/staff-living-with-nursing-home-residents-with-covid-19-reduced-deaths-cases-study/

11 — Risks to the Elderly Living Inside vs Outside Institutional Settings

Government of Canada. (2021, May 8). *(COVID-19) daily epidemiology update*. Retrieved from https://web.archive.org/web/20210509074839if_/https://health-infobase.canada.ca/covid-19/epidemiological-summary-covid-19-cases.html

Statistics Canada. (2020, July 1). Population estimates on July 1st, by age and sex. *Statistics Canada.* Retrieved from https://www150.statcan.gc.ca/t1/tbl1/en/tv.action?pid=1710 000501&pickMembers%5B0%5D=1.11&pickMembers%5B1 %5D=2.1&cubeTimeFrame.startYear=2016&cubeTimeFrame. endYear=2020&referencePeriods=20160101%2C20200101

Library of Parliament (2020, October 22). Long-term Care Homes in Canada – How are they Funded and Regulated. *Hill Notes.* Retrieved from https://hillnotes.ca/2020/10/22/long-term-care-homes-in-canada-how-are-they-funded-and-regulated/#:~:text=According%20to%20census%20data%2C %20almost,(LTC)%20facilities%20in%202016.

Ruechel, J. (2021, January 25). Bystander at the Switch: The Moral Case Against COVID Lockdowns. *www.juliusruechel.com.* Retrieved from https://www.juliusruechel.com/2021/01/bystander-at-switch-moral-case-against.html

Malakieh, J. (2020, December 21). Adult and youth correctional statistics in Canada, 2018/2019. *Statistics Canada.* Retrieved from https://www150.statcan.gc.ca/n1/pub/85-002-x/2020001/article/00016-eng.htm

The Conversation (2018, July 6). Pre-existing conditions, the age group most vulnerable if coverage goes away. *The Conversation.* Retrieved from https://theconversation.com/pre-existing-conditions-the-age-group-most-vulnerable-if-coverage-goes-away-98442

Canadian Institute for Health Information. (2011, January). Seniors and the Health Care System: What is the Impact of Multiple Chronic Conditions? *CIHI.* Retrieved from https://secure.cihi.ca/free_products/air-chronic_disease_aib_en.pdf

Modiga et al. (2021, March 17). Excess mortality for men and women above age 70 according to level of care during the first wave of COVID-19 pandemic in Sweden: A population-based study. *The Lancet Regional Health – Europe.* Retrieved from https://www.thelancet.com/action/showPdf?pii=S2666-7762%2821%2900049-1

12 — Let's Bring in the Rest of the Data

Ireton, J. (2021, March 30). Canada's nursing homes have worst records for COVID-19 deaths among wealthy nations: report. *CBC News.* Retrieved from https://www.cbc.ca/news/canada/ottawa/canada-record-covid-19-deaths-wealthy-countries-cihi-1.5968749

13 — Honest Numbers, Dishonest Health Officials, and a Blatant Disregard for the Rules

Dr. Theresa Tam. (2020, January 29). *HESA Committee Meeting Minutes.* Retrieved from House of Commons of Canada - Standing Committee on Health (HESA): https://www.ourcommons.ca/DocumentViewer/en/43-1/HESA/meeting-1/evidence

WHO (2019, November 19). Global Influenza Programme. *Non-pharmaceutical public health measures for mitigating the risk and impact of epidemic and pandemic influenza.* Retrieved from https://apps.who.int/iris/bitstream/handle/10665/329438/9789241516839-eng.pdf?ua=1

@Milhouse_Van_Ho. (2021, May 14). Mortality in Canada (thread). *Twitter.* Retrieved from https://twitter.com/Milhouse_Van_Ho/status/1393213483550978057

Ruechel, J. (2021, January 25). Bystander at the Switch: The Moral Case Against COVID Lockdowns. *www.juliusruechel.com.* Retrieved from https://www.juliusruechel.com/2021/01/bystander-at-switch-moral-case-against.html

Statistics Canada. (2020, November 26). Deaths, by month. *Statistics Canada*. Retrieved from https://www150.statcan.gc.ca/t1/tbl1/en/tv.action?pid=1310 070801

Johansen, N. (2021, May 21). Half of deaths unvaccinated. *Castanet News*. Retrieved from https://www.castanet.net/news/Kelowna/334701/Half-of-the-those-who-died-at-Spring-Valley-not-vaccinated

@TOPublicHealth (2020, June 24). Individuals who have died with COVID-19, but not as a result of COVID-19 are included in the case counts for COVID-19 deaths in Toronto. *Toronto Public Health on Twitter*. Retrieved from https://twitter.com/TOPublicHealth/status/12758883900602 85967

@Milhouse_Van_Ho. (2021, May 14). Mortality in Canada (thread). *Twitter*. Retrieved from https://twitter.com/Milhouse_Van_Ho/status/139321348355 0978057

Furey, A. (2021, May 21). FUREY: Fewer Canadian kids hospitalized with COVID than previously thought, report shows. *Toronto Sun*. Retrieved from https://torontosun.com/news/national/furey-fewer-canadian-kids-hospitalized-with-covid-than-previously-thought-report-shows

Furey, A. (2021, May 21). FUREY: Fewer Canadian kids hospitalized with COVID than previously thought, report shows. *Toronto Sun*. Retrieved from https://torontosun.com/news/national/furey-fewer-canadian-kids-hospitalized-with-covid-than-previously-thought-report-shows

@Milhouse_Van_Ho. (2021, May 14). Mortality in Canada (thread). *Twitter*. Retrieved from https://twitter.com/Milhouse_Van_Ho/status/139321348355 0978057

References

Statistics Canada. (2020, November 26). Deaths, by month. *Statistics Canada*. Retrieved from https://www150.statcan.gc.ca/t1/tbl1/en/tv.action?pid=1310 070801

Ruechel, J. (2021, January 25). Bystander at the Switch: The Moral Case Against COVID Lockdowns. *www.juliusruechel.com*. Retrieved from https://www.juliusruechel.com/2021/01/bystander-at-switch-moral-case-against.html

The Canadian Press. (2021, March 31). The flu season that never was: COVID-19 pandemic keeps other viruses at bay. *CTV News*. Retrieved from https://www.ctvnews.ca/health/coronavirus/the-flu-season-that-never-was-covid-19-pandemic-keeps-other-viruses-at-bay-1.5369864

Wu et al. (2020, September 4). Interference between rhinovirus and influenza A virus: a clinical data analysis and experimental infection study. *The Lancet*. Retrieved from https://www.thelancet.com/journals/lanmic/article/PIIS2666-5247(20)30114-2/fulltext?s=09

Schultz-Cherry, S. (2015, May 5). Viral Interference: The Case of Influenza Viruses. *Oxford Academic: The Journal of Infectious Diseases*. Retrieved from https://academic.oup.com/jid/article/212/11/1690/2911897

Nickbakhsh et al. (2019, December 26). Virus-virus interactions impact the population dynamics of influenza and the common cold. *PNAS*. Retrieved from https://www.pnas.org/content/116/52/27142

Government of Canada. (2021, June 3). Respiratory Virus Detections in Canada. *Government of Canada*. Retrieved from https://www.canada.ca/en/public-health/services/surveillance/respiratory-virus-detections-canada.html

Tam, T. MD. (2021, May 14). COVID-19 key concerns in Canada: it's all down to maintaining the great progress we are making! *Twitter*. Retrieved from https://twitter.com/Milhouse_Van_Ho/status/139321348355 0978057

Rayner, G. (2021, May 14). Use of fear to control behavior in covid crisis was 'totalitarian', admits scientists. *The Telegraph*. Retrieved from https://www.telegraph.co.uk/news/2021/05/14/scientists-admit-totalitarian-use-fear-control-behaviour-covid/

@abirballan. (2021, May 21). 'Scientists on a committee that encouraged the use of fear to control people's behavior during the Covid pandemic have admitted its work was 'unethical' and 'totalitarian'. *Twitter*. Retrieved from https://twitter.com/abirballan/status/1395975768363216896

14 — How Lockdowns Bring Death to the Vulnerable

Our World in Data. (2021, March 17). Daily new COVID-19 deaths by per million people. *Our World in Data.org*. Retrieved from https://ourworldindata.org/covid-deaths

Smith, A.K., DR, MS, MPH., Kelly, A. MSW. (2010, August 4). Social Support is Key to Nursing Home Length of Stay Before Death. *UCSF*. Retrieved from https://www.ucsf.edu/news/2010/08/98172/social-support-key-nursing-home-length-stay-death

Jones, A. M. (2020, November 19). Facing another retirement home lockdown, 90-year-old chooses medically assisted death. *CTV News*. Retrieved from https://www.ctvnews.ca/health/facing-another-retirement-home-lockdown-90-year-old-chooses-medically-assisted-death-1.5197140

Supreme Court of Canada. (1986). The Oakes Test. *Center for Constitutional Studies.* Retrieved from https://www.constitutionalstudies.ca/2019/07/oakes-test/

15 — The Price of Fear

WHO (2019, November 19). Global Influenza Programme. *Non-pharmaceutical public health measures for mitigating the risk and impact of epidemic and pandemic influenza.* Retrieved from https://apps.who.int/iris/bitstream/handle/10665/329438/9 789241516839-eng.pdf?ua=1

Ruechel, J. (2020, September 29). Droplets and Aerosols, Why Catching the Sneeze Doesn't Reduce Viral Transmission. *www.juliusruechel.com.* Retrieved from https://www.juliusruechel.com/2020/09/droplets-and-aerosols-why-catching.html

Gray, W. (2020, March 30). Canada's top Doctor says wearing a mask is not recommended. *My Grand Prairie Now.* Retrieved from https://www.mygrandeprairienow.com/68624/canadas-top-doctor-says-wearing-a-mask-is-not-recommended/

Derfel, A. (2020, April 8). Public health, Police find bodies, feces at Dorval seniors' residence: sources. *Montreal Gazette.* Retrieved from https://web.archive.org/web/20200415022629if_/https://mo ntrealgazette.com/news/local-news/public-health-police-find-bodies-feces-at-dorval-seniors-residence-sources/

Ruechel, J. (2020, September 29). *Opinion is Not Evidence, Ignoring Science to Follow Gut Instinct.* www.juliusruechel.com. Retrieved from https://www.juliusruechel.com/2020/09/opinion-is-not-evidence-ignoring.html

Public Health Agency of Canada. (2020, March 19). Coronavirus disease (COVID-19): Prevention and Risks. *Government of Canada.* Retrieved from https://web.archive.org/web/20200320001728if_/https://ww

w.canada.ca/en/public-health/services/diseases/2019-novel-coronavirus-infection/prevention-risks.html

Swiss Policy Research. (2020, July 25). *Tönnies: Corona-Ausbruch trotz Maskenpflicht. Fakten zu Covid-19.* Retrieved from https://swprs.org/tonnies-corona-ausbruch-trotz-maskenpflicht/

Wikipedia. (2019, December). Diamond Princess (ship). *Wikipedia.* Retrieved from https://en.wikipedia.org/wiki/Diamond_Princess_(ship)

Berlan, J.M. (2020, July 26). "Eliminating staff 'cross-traffic' could have cut nursing home COVID-19 deaths by 44 percent, researchers find. *McKnight's Long-Term Care News.* Retrieved from https://www.mcknights.com/news/researchers-find-how-44-percent-of-nursing-covid-19-deaths-could-be-prevented/

Brown, D. (2020, August 18). Staff living with nursing home residents with COVID-19 reduced deaths, cases: study. *McKnight's Long-Term Care News.* Retrieved from https://www.mcknights.com/news/staff-living-with-nursing-home-residents-with-covid-19-reduced-deaths-cases-study/

Almilaji, O. (2020, December 30). Air Recirculation Role in the spread of COVID-19 Onboard the Diamond Princess Cruise Ship during a Quarantine Period. *Aerosol and Air Quality Research.* Retrieved from https://aaqr.org/articles/aaqr-20-07-covid-0495

Mousavi et al. (2020, August 13). Performance analysis of portable HEPA filters and temporary plastic anterooms on the spread of surrogate coronavirus. *PMC US National Library of Medicine National Institute of Health.* Retrieved from https://www.ncbi.nlm.nih.gov/pmc/articles/PMC7424318/

Frey, N. (2020, March 20). Do HEPA air purifiers filter out the COVID-19 virus? *Vaniman.* Retrieved from https://www.vaniman.com/do-hepa-air-purifiers-filter-out-the-covid-19-virus/

Howlett, K. (2021, April 22). Ontario hospitals transfer patients to long-term care to free up beds for COVID patients. *The Globe and Mail* Retrieved from https://www.theglobeandmail.com/canada/article-ontario-hospitals-transfer-patients-to-long-term-care-to-free-up-beds/

Trinh, J. (2021, May 18). CHEO could turn to adult hospitals as mental health cases surge. CBC. Retrieved from https://www.cbc.ca/news/canada/ottawa/cheo-ottawa-mental-health-children-1.6029936

Statistics Canada. (2020, March 10). Provisional death counts and excess mortality, January to December 2020. *The Daily*. Retrieved from https://web.archive.org/web/20210412213538if_/https://www150.statcan.gc.ca/n1/daily-quotidien/210310/dq210310c-eng.htm

Lowrie, M. (2021, February 7). Doctors fear an impending wave of cancer patients after COVID-19 delays. *Terrace Standard*. Retrieved from https://www.terracestandard.com/news/doctors-fear-an-impending-wave-of-cancer-patients-after-covid-19-delays/

Beasley, D. (2020, September 17). WFP Chief warns of grave dangers of economic impact of Coronavirus as millions are pushed further into hunger. *World Food Programme*. Retrieved from https://www.wfp.org/news/wfp-chief-warns-grave-dangers-economic-impact-coronavirus-millions-are-pushed-further-hunger

16 — The Opportunity Cost of Waiting for a Vaccine and Ignoring Pandemic Planning Guidelines

Government of Ontario. (2021, June 9). Roadmap to reopen – key highlights. *Government of Ontario*. Retrieved from https://www.ontario.ca/page/reopening-ontario

Lundgren J.D. (2021, February 18). National Cohort Study of Effectiveness and Safety of SARS-CoV-2/COVID-19 Vaccines (ENFORCE)(ENFORCE). *NIH U.S. National Library of Medicine*. Retrieved from https://clinicaltrials.gov/ct2/show/NCT04760132

British Medical Journal. (1996, December 7). Permissible Medical Experiments. *The Nuremberg Code (1947)*. Retrieved from https://clinicaltrials.gov/ct2/show/NCT04760132

17 — Is Informed Consent Even Possible for People Who Already Have Herd Immunity? Implications of the Nuremberg Code.

OpenVAERS (n.d.) *COVID Vaccine Adverse Event Reports Through May 14th, 2020,* Retrieved from: https://openvaers.com/index.php

VAERS (n.d.) *The Vaccine Adverse Event Reporting System (VAERS).* Search Query on May 14th, 2021. Retrieved from: https://wonder.cdc.gov/vaers.html

Health Day News. (2021, March 17). *COVID-19 Antibodies Found in One in Five U.S. Blood Donations.* Retrieved from Health Day News: https://consumer.healthday.com/covid-19-antibodies-found-in-one-in-five-u-s-blood-donations-2651116864.html

Majdoubi et al. (2021, March 15). A majority of uninfected adults show preexisting antibody reactivity against SARS-CoV-2. *JCI Insight*, 6(8), e146316. Retrieved from JCI Insight: https://insight.jci.org/articles/view/146316

Nelde et al., (2020, June 17). *SARS-CoV-2 T-cell epitopes define heterologous and COVID-19-induced T-cell recognition.* Research Square. Retrieved from: https://www.researchsquare.com/article/rs-35331/v1

Swiss Policy Research. (2020, September). *Facts about Covid-19 (archive).* Retrieved from Swiss Policy Research: https://swprs.org/facts-about-covid-19-archive/

CNBC Health and Science. (2020, October 5). *WHO says 10% of global population may have been infected with virus.* Retrieved from CNBC Health and Science: https://www.cnbc.com/2020/10/05/who-10percent-of-worlds-people-may-have-been-infected-with-virus-.html

18 — Bypassing Parental Guardianship – Do Children Really Understand Their Risks Without Parental Oversight?

Judd, A, (2021, May 20). B.C. Youth who want the COVID-19 vaccine do not need parental consent or a signed form. *Global News.* Retrieved from https://globalnews.ca/news/7881765/bc-covid-19-vaccine-youth-consent-infants-act/

City of Toronto. (2021, May 1). City of Toronto vaccination clinic appointments opening to youth aged 12 and older starting this Sunday. *@cityoftoronto on Twitter.* Retrieved from https://twitter.com/cityoftoronto/status/139585707731524403
2

B.C. Center for Disease Control. (2018, May). The Infants Act, Mature Minor Consent and Immunization. *HealthLinkBC File Number: 119.* Retrieved from https://www.healthlinkbc.ca/healthlinkbc-files/infants-act-mature-minor-consent-and-immunization

B.C. Center for Disease Control. (2018, May). The Infants Act, Mature Minor Consent and Immunization. *HealthLinkBC File Number: 119.* Retrieved from https://www.healthlinkbc.ca/healthlinkbc-files/infants-act-mature-minor-consent-and-immunization

Government of Saskatchewan. (2021, May 20). Vaccination Details for Youth 12+. *Health Care Administration and Provider Resources.* Retrieved from https://www.saskatchewan.ca/government/health-care-administration-and-provider-resources/treatment-procedures-and-guidelines/emerging-public-health-issues/2019-novel-coronavirus/covid-19-vaccine/vaccine-delivery-phases/vaccination-details-for-youth

Schneebaum, G. (2015, Spring). What is Wrong with Sex in Authority Relations? A Study in Law and Social Theory. *Journal of Criminal Law and Criminology, 105(2)*. Retrieved from https://scholarlycommons.law.northwestern.edu/cgi/viewcontent.cgi?article=7559&context=jclc

19 — When Government Goes "All-In" on One Strategy, All Others Are Put Aside. The Sorry Tale of Ivermectin and its Unpopular Friends

U.S. Food and Drug Administration. (2020, November 20). *Emergency Use Authorization for Vaccines Explained.* Retrieved from https://www.fda.gov/vaccines-blood-biologics/vaccines/emergency-use-authorization-vaccines-explained

Ivmmeta.com (Version 83). (2021, May 18). *Ivermectin for COVID-19: real-time meta-analysis of 60 studies.* Retrieved from https://ivmmeta.com/

Ivmmeta.com (Version 83). (2021, May 18). *Ivermectin for COVID-19: real-time meta-analysis of 60 studies.* Retrieved from https://ivmmeta.com/

Government of Canada. (2021, January 29). *Remdesivir (Veklury): What you should know.* Government of Canada. Retrieved from https://web.archive.org/web/20210312075401if_/https://www.canada.ca/en/health-canada/services/drugs-health-products/covid19-industry/drugs-vaccines-treatments/treatments/remdesivir.html

CATIE News. (2020, August 6). Remdesivir (Veklury) – The first drug approved in Canada for COVID-19 treatment. *CATIE News.* Retrieved from https://www.catie.ca/en/catienews/2020-08-06/remdesivir-veklury-first-drug-approved-canada-covid-19-treatment

BC Center for Disease Control. (2021, April 9). *Treatments.* Provincial Health Services Authority. Retrieved from https://web.archive.org/web/20210422161148/http://www.bccdc.ca/health-professionals/clinical-resources/covid-19-care/clinical-care/treatments

Farley, R. (2021, January 12). How much does ivermectin cost? Can we expect shortages due to coronavirus? *Pharmacy Checker.com.* Retrieved from https://www.pharmacychecker.com/askpc/ivermectin-cost-insurance/

Ivmmeta.com (Version 83). (2021, May 18). *Ivermectin for COVID-19: real-time meta-analysis of 60 studies.* Retrieved from https://ivmmeta.com/

7UMMIT Magazine. (2021, April 23). Canadian Health Minister Dismisses Peer-Reviewed Studies on Vitamin D as 'Fake News'. *7UMMIT Magazine on YouTube.* Retrieved from https://youtu.be/-SCAZEEYSTs

Zhou et al., (2018, August). Preventive Effects of Vitamin D on Seasonal Influenza A in Infants: A Multicenter, Randomized, Open, Controlled Clinical Trial. *The Pediatric Infectious Disease Journal, 37(8), 749-754.* Retrieved from https://journals.lww.com/pidj/fulltext/2018/08000/preventive_effects_of_vitamin_d_on_seasonal.5.aspx

BBC News. (2020, November 28). Covid: Free Vitamin D pills for 2.5 million vulnerable in England. *BBC News.* Retrieved from https://www.bbc.com/news/health-55108613

20 — The Lies… Summary

Jones, A.M. (2020, November 19). Facing another retirement home lockdown, 90-year-old chooses medically assisted death. *CTV*

News. Retrieved from https://www.bbc.com/news/health-55108613

21 — George Washington's Gamble

Swiss Policy Research. (2021, September). *Studies on Covid Lethality.* Retrieved from Swiss Policy Research: https://swprs.org/studies-on-covid-19-lethality/

Thaker, B. (n.d.). *Disease in the Revolutionary War.* The Washington Library. Retrieved from George Washington's Mount Vernon: https://www.mountvernon.org/library/digitalhistory/digital-encyclopedia/article/disease-in-the-revolutionary-war/

Thaker, B. (n.d.). *Disease in the Revolutionary War.* The Washington Library. Retrieved from George Washington's Mount Vernon: https://www.mountvernon.org/library/digitalhistory/digital-encyclopedia/article/disease-in-the-revolutionary-war/

22 — Calculating Your Vegas Odds

CDC. (n.d.). *Overview, History, and How the Safety Process Works.* Retrieved September 23, 2021, from Centers for Disease Control and Prevention (CDC). Retrieved on June 15th, 2021: https://www.cdc.gov/vaccinesafety/ensuringsafety/history/index.html

23 — The Calculations: Vegas Odds of Death from Covid

CDC. (2021, March 19). *COVID-19 Pandemic Planning Scenarios.* Retrieved June 7, 2021, from Centers for Disease Control and Prevention: https://web.archive.org/web/20210607143315/https://www.cdc.gov/coronavirus/2019-ncov/hcp/planning-scenarios.html

Swiss Policy Research. (2020, September). *Facts about Covid-19 (archive).* Retrieved from Swiss Policy Research: https://swprs.org/facts-about-covid-19-archive/

References

Majdoubi et al. (2021, March 15). A majority of uninfected adults show preexisting antibody reactivity against SARS-CoV-2. *JCI Insight*, 6(8), e146316. Retrieved from JCI Insight: https://insight.jci.org/articles/view/146316

Doshi, P. (2020, September 17). Covid-19: Do many people have pre-existing immunity? *The British Medical Journal*, 370, m3563. Retrieved from: https://www.bmj.com/content/370/bmj.m3563

O'Brien et al. (2020, November 16). *COVID-19 death comorbidities in Canada*. Statistics Canada. Retrieved from: https://web.archive.org/web/20210219195135if_/https://www150.statcan.gc.ca/n1/pub/45-28-0001/2020001/article/00087-eng.htm

Agency for Healthcare Research and Quality. (2014, April). *Multiple Chronic Conditions Chartbook: 2010 Medical Expenditure Panel Survey Data*. Retrieved from Agency for Healthcare Research and Quality: https://www.ahrq.gov/sites/default/files/wysiwyg/professionals/prevention-chronic-care/decision/mcc/mccchartbook.pdf

Gao et al. (2021, June 1). Associations between body-mass index and COVID-19 severity in 6·9 million people in England: a prospective, community-based, cohort study. *The Lancet Diabetes & Endocrinology*, 9(6), P350-359. Retrieved from The Lancet Diabetes & Endocrinology: https://www.thelancet.com/journals/landia/article/PIIS2213-8587(21)00089-9/fulltext

Gao et al. (2021, June 1). Supplementary appendix. Associations between body-mass index and COVID-19 severity in 6·9 million people in England: a prospective, community-based, cohort study. *The Lancet Diabetes & Endocrinology*, 9(6), P350-359. Retrieved from The Lancet Diabetes & Endocrinology: https://www.thelancet.com/cms/10.1016/S2213-8587(21)00089-9/attachment/88cb76d8-d2d5-4b73-9a05-fffefad4de8d/mmc1.pdf

Gao et al. (2021, June 1). Supplementary appendix. Associations between body-mass index and COVID-19 severity in 6·9 million people in England: a prospective, community-based, cohort study. *The Lancet Diabetes & Endocrinology,* 9(6), P350-359. Retrieved from The Lancet Diabetes & Endocrinology: https://www.thelancet.com/cms/10.1016/S2213-8587(21)00089-9/attachment/88cb76d8-d2d5-4b73-9a05-fffefad4de8d/mmc1.pdf

24 — The Calculations: Vegas Odds of Death or Injury from the Vaccines

Medicines and Healthcare products Regulatory Agency (MHRA GOV.UK). (n.d.). *Yellow Card.* Retrieved from Yellow Card Adverse Drug Reactions: https://yellowcard.mhra.gov.uk/

Lawrie, T. (2021, June 9). *Urgent preliminary report of Yellow Card data up to 26th May 2021.* Retrieved from Evidence-based Medicine Consultancy Ltd: https://b3d2650e-e929-4448-a527-4eeb59304c7f.filesusr.com/ugd/593c4f_b2acdef3774b4e9ca06e9fae526fd5cd.pdf

Lawrie, T. (2021, June 9). *Urgent preliminary report of Yellow Card data up to 26th May 2021.* Retrieved from Evidence-based Medicine Consultancy Ltd: https://b3d2650e-e929-4448-a527-4eeb59304c7f.filesusr.com/ugd/593c4f_b2acdef3774b4e9ca06e9fae526fd5cd.pdf

CDC. (2021, June 9). *Vaccine Adverse Event Reporting System (VAERS).* Retrieved June 9, 2021, from Centers for Disease Control and Prevention (CDC): https://wonder.cdc.gov/vaers.html

25 — Vegas Odds Discussion

CDC. (2021, June 9). *Vaccine Adverse Event Reporting System (VAERS).* Retrieved June 9, 2021, from Centers for Disease

Control and Prevention (CDC):
https://wonder.cdc.gov/vaers.html

Semba, R. (2004, March 1). Measles blindness. *Public Health and the Eye*, 49(2), P243-255. Retrieved from https://www.surveyophthalmol.com/article/S0039-6257(03)00179-6/fulltext

Wikipedia. (n.d.). *Antibody-dependent enhancement.* Retrieved on June 24, 2021, from Wikipedia: https://en.wikipedia.org/wiki/Antibody-dependent_enhancement

27 — You Don't Need a Knight in Shining Armour to Ride to Granny's Rescue When She Can Have Her Own Sherman Tank

WHO (2019, November 19). Global Influenza Programme. *Non-pharmaceutical public health measures for mitigating the risk and impact of epidemic and pandemic influenza.* Retrieved from https://apps.who.int/iris/bitstream/handle/10665/329438/9789241516839-eng.pdf?ua=1

29 — Viral Reservoirs: The Fantasy of Eradication

Russell, Clark Donald. (2011, October 10). Eradicating Infectious Disease: Can We and Should We? *Frontiers in Immunology.* Retrieved from https://www.ncbi.nlm.nih.gov/pmc/articles/PMC3341977/

Maron, Dina Fine. (2021, August 2). Wild U.S. Found with Coronavirus Antibodies. *National Geographic.* Retrieved from https://www.nationalgeographic.com/animals/article/wild-us-deer-found-with-coronavirus-antibodies?irgwc=1&irclickid=zj5yOKVyZxyORwZwUx0Mo38qUkBRHUUeXyFWzc0&cmpid=org%3Dngp%3A%3Amc%3Daffiliate%3A%3Asrc%3Daffiliate%3A%3Acmp%3Dsubs_aff%3A%3Aadd%3DSkimbit%20Ltd.

Mallapaty, Smriti. (2021, August 2). The coronavirus is rife in common US deer. *Nature.* Retrieved from https://www.nature.com/articles/d41586-021-02110-8?utm_medium=affiliate&utm_source=commission_junction &utm_campaign=3_nsn6445_deeplink_PID100093539&utm_ content=deeplink

Mallapaty, Smriti. (2021, August 2). The search for animals harbouring coronavirus – and why it matters. *Nature.* Retrieved from https://www.nature.com/articles/d41586-021-02110-8?utm_medium=affiliate&utm_source=commission_junction &utm_campaign=3_nsn6445_deeplink_PID100093539&utm_ content=deeplink

30 — SARS: The Exception to the Rule?

Gorvett, Zaria. (2020, September 28). The deadly viruses that vanished without trace. *BBC.com.* Retrieved from https://www.bbc.com/future/article/20200918-why-some-deadly-viruses-vanish-and-go-extinct

WHO (2019, November 19). Global Influenza Programme. *Non-pharmaceutical public health measures for mitigating the risk and impact of epidemic and pandemic influenza.* Retrieved from https://apps.who.int/iris/bitstream/handle/10665/329438/9 789241516839-eng.pdf?ua=1

31 — Fast Mutations: The Fantasy of Control through Herd Immunity

Wikipedia. (n.d.). Respiratory syncytial virus. *Wikipedia.* Retrieved on August 31, 2021, from: https://en.wikipedia.org/wiki/Respiratory_syncytial_virus

Science Daily. (2015, May 21). Why you need one vaccine for measles and many for the flu. *Science News.* Retrieved from

https://www.sciencedaily.com/releases/2015/05/1505211336
28.htm

33 — Spiked: The Fantasy of Preventing Infection

Doshi, Peter, senior editor. (2021, August 23). Does the FDA think
these data justify the first full approval of a covid-19 vaccine?
The British Medical Journal. Retrieved from
https://blogs.bmj.com/bmj/2021/08/23/does-the-fda-think-
these-data-justify-the-first-full-approval-of-a-covid-19-vaccine/

34 — Antibodies, B-Cells and T-Cells: Why Immunity to Respiratory Viruses Fades So Quickly

Cohen, Jon. (2019, April 18). How long do vaccines last? The
surprising answers may help protect people longer. *Science.org.*
Retrieved from
https://www.science.org/news/2019/04/how-long-do-
vaccines-last-surprising-answers-may-help-protect-people-
longer

Simpson, Brain W. (2021, May 28). Why COVID-19 Vaccines
Offer better Protection Than Infection. *Johns Hopkins Blomberg
School of Public Health.* Retrieved from
https://web.archive.org/web/20210528162934/https:/www.j
hsph.edu/covid-19/articles/why-covid-19-vaccines-offer-
better-protection-than-infection.html

Holmes, Kathryn V. (2003, June 1). SARS coronavirus: a new
challenge for prevention and therapy. *The Journal of Clinical
Investigation.* Retrieved from
https://www.bbc.com/news/health-55108613

Saif, Linda J. (2010, July 1). Bovine respiratory coronavirus.
ScienceDirect, 26(2), 349-364. Retrieved from
https://www.sciencedirect.com/science/article/pii/S0749072
010000113?via%3Dihub

Saif, Linda J. (2020, March 24). Vaccines for COVID-19: Perspectives, Prospects, and Challenges Based on Candidate SARS, MERS, and Animal Coronavirus Vaccines. *European Medical Journal (EMJ)*. Retrieved from: https://www.emjreviews.com/allergy-immunology/article/vaccines-for-covid-19-perspectives-prospects-and-challenges-based-on-candidate-sars-mers-and-animal-coronavirus-vaccines/

Wu et al. (2007, October). Duration of Antibody Responses after Severe Acute Respiratory Syndrome. *Emerging Infectious Diseases Journal*. (13(10) 1562-1564. Retrieved from the Centers for Disease Control and Prevention: https://wwwnc.cdc.gov/eid/article/13/10/07-0576_article

Alshukairi, Abeer N. (2021, May). Longevity of Middle East Respiratory Syndrome Coronavirus Antibody Responses in Humans, Saudi Arabia. *Emerging Infectious Diseases Journal* 27(5). 1472-1476. Retrieved from the Center for Disease Control and Prevention. https://wwwnc.cdc.gov/eid/article/27/5/20-4056_article#:~:text=In%20conclusion%2C%20we%20showed%20that,durable%20immunity%20against%20the%20virus.

Swiss Policy Research. (2021, August 20). *Covid Vaccines: The Good, The Bad, The Ugly*. Retrieved from Swiss Policy Research: https://swprs.org/covid-vaccines-the-good-the-bad-the-ugly/

35 — Manufacturing Dangerous Variants: Lessons from the 1918 Spanish Flu

Swiss Policy Research. (2021, August 20). *Covid Vaccines: A Shot in the Dark?* Retrieved from Swiss Policy Research: https://swprs.org/covid-vaccines-a-shot-in-the-dark/

Roos, Dave. (2010, December 22). Why the Second Wave of the 1918 Flu Pandemic Was So Deadly. *History Channel*. Retrieved from History Stories:

https://www.history.com/news/spanish-flu-second-wave-resurgence

36 — Leaky Vaccines, Antibody-Dependent Enhancement, and the Marek Effect

Financial Times. (2021, August 23). Israel hopes boosters can avert new lockdown as COVID vaccine efficacy fades. Retrieved from https://www.ft.com/content/23cdbf8c-b5ef-4596-bb46-f510606ab556

Armour, Stephanie and Hopkins, Jared S. (2021, August 26). Biden Administration Likely to Approve Covid-19 Boosters at Six Months. *The Wall Street Journal.* Retrieved from https://www.wsj.com/articles/biden-administration-plans-covid-19-vaccine-boosters-at-six-months-instead-of-eight-11629919356

Wingrove, Josh and Jacobs, Jennifer (2021, August 27). Biden Weighs Speeding Up Booster-Shot Timeline by 3 Months. *Bloomberg.* Retrieved from https://www.bloomberg.com/news/articles/2021-08-27/biden-says-u-s-considering-starting-booster-shots-earlier-ksujzrim

Dinerstein, Chuck MD, MBA. (2018, October 26). Influenza Vaccination Is Global, But Not the Same. *American Council on Science and Health.* Retrieved from https://www.acsh.org/news/2018/10/26/influenza-vaccination-global-not-same-12504

Akpan, Nskikan. (2015, July 27). This chicken vaccine makes its virus more dangerous. *PBS Science.* Retrieved from https://www.acsh.org/news/2018/10/26/influenza-vaccination-global-not-same-12504

eugyppius. (2021, Aug 11). The Marek Effect. *Marek's disease is caused by an alphaherpesvirus that infects poultry.* Retrieved from https://eugyppius.substack.com/p/the-marek-effect

Yahi et al. (2021, August 9). Infection-enhancing anti-SARS-CoV-2 antibodies recognize both the original Wuhan/D614G strain and Delta variants. A potential risk for mass vaccination? *Journal of Infection.* Retrieved from https://www.journalofinfection.com/article/S0163-4453(21)00392-3/fulltext

Wikipedia. (n.d.). Antibody-dependent enhancement. *Wikipedia.* Retrieved from Wikipedia on August 4, 2021: https://en.wikipedia.org/wiki/Antibody-dependent_enhancement

Su, Shan, Du, Lanying, and Jiang, Shibo. (2020, October 16). Learning from the past: development of safe and effective COVID-19 vaccines. *Nature reviews microbiology.* 19. 211-219. Retrieved from https://www.nature.com/articles/s41579-020-00462-y

Su, Shan, Du, Lanying, and Jiang, Shibo. (2020, October 16). Learning from the past: development of safe and effective COVID-19 vaccines. *Nature reviews microbiology.* 19. 211-219. Retrieved from https://www.nature.com/articles/s41579-020-00462-y

Open VAERS. (2021, August 20). Reports from the Vaccine Adverse Events Reporting System. *VAERS COVID Vaccine Data.* Retrieved from https://www.openvaers.com/covid-data

37 — Anti-Virus Security Updates: Cross-Reactive Immunity Through Repeated Exposure

Huang et al. (2020, September 17). A systematic review of antibody mediated immunity to coronaviruses: kinetics, correlates of protection, and association with severity. *Nature Communications.* 11. 4704. Retrieved from https://www.nature.com/articles/s41467-020-18450-4

Majdoubi et al. (2021, March 15). A majority of uninfected adults show preexisting antibody reactivity against SARS-CoV-2. *JCI*

Insight, 6(8), e146316. Retrieved from JCI Insight: https://insight.jci.org/articles/view/146316

38 — The Not-So-Novel Virus: The *Diamond Princess* Cruise Ship Outbreak Proved We Have Cross-Reactive Immunity

Tasker, John Paul. (2021, August 13). Federal government to require vaccinations for all federal public servants, air and train passengers. *CBC News*. https://www.cbc.ca/news/politics/federal-government-mandatory-vaccinations-1.6140131

Ioannidis, John P.A. (2020, March 17). A fiasco in the making? As the coronavirus pandemic takes hold, we are making decisions without reliable data. *STAT News*. Retrieved from https://www.statnews.com/2020/03/17/a-fiasco-in-the-making-as-the-coronavirus-pandemic-takes-hold-we-are-making-decisions-without-reliable-data/

Plucinski et al. (2021, May 18). Coronavirus Disease 2019 (COVID-19) in Americans Aboard the Diamond Princess Cruise Ship. *National Library of Medicine*. 72(10). 448-457 Retrieved from https://pubmed.ncbi.nlm.nih.gov/32785683/

National Institute of Infectious Diseases, Japan. (2019, February 19). Field Briefing: Diamond Princess COVID-19 Cases. *NIID*. Retrieved from https://www.niid.go.jp/niid/en/2019-ncov-e/9407-covid-dp-fe-01.html

Alpsdake. (2019, December 8). Diamond Princess seen from Mount Asama around port of Toba in Toba, Mie Prefecture, Japan. CC BY-SA 4.0. Retrieved from *Wikimedia Commons*: https://en.wikipedia.org/wiki/COVID-19_pandemic_on_Diamond_Princess#/media/File:Diamond_Princess_(ship,_2004)_-_cropped.jpg

Majdoubi et al. (2021, March 15). A majority of uninfected adults show preexisting antibody reactivity against SARS-CoV-2. JCI

Insight, 6(8), e146316. Retrieved from JCI Insight: https://insight.jci.org/articles/view/146316

Beretta, Alberto; Cranage, Martin; and Zipeto, Donato. (2020, October 15). Is Cross-Reactive Immunity Triggering COVID-19 Immunopathogenesis? *Frontiers in Immunology*. Retrieved from https://www.frontiersin.org/articles/10.3389/fimmu.2020.567710/full

Wikipedia. (n.d.). Operation Warp Speed. *Wikipedia*. Retrieved on August 31, 2021, from https://en.wikipedia.org/wiki/Operation_Warp_Speed

39 — Mother Knows Best: Vitamin D, Playing in Puddles, and Sweaters

Harvard Health Publishing. (2010, January 1). Out in the cold. *Harvard Medical School*. Retrieved from https://www.health.harvard.edu/staying-healthy/out-in-the-cold

Canadian Health Minister Patty Hajdu. (2021, April 23). Canadian Health Minister Dismisses Peer-Reviewed Studies on Vitamin D as 'Fake News'. 7UMMIT Magazine *YouTube Channel*. Retrieved from YouTube: https://www.youtube.com/watch?v=-SCAZEEYSTs

40 — The Paradox: Why COVID-Zero Makes People More Vulnerability to Other Viruses

McClure, Tess. (2021, July 8). New Zealand children falling ill in high numbers due to Covid 'immunity debt'. *The Guardian*. Retrieved from https://www.theguardian.com/world/2021/jul/08/new-zealand-children-falling-ill-in-high-numbers-due-to-covid-immunity-debt

McClure, Tess. (2021, July 8). New Zealand children falling ill in high numbers due to Covid 'immunity debt'. *The Guardian*. Retrieved from https://www.theguardian.com/world/2021/jul/08/new-zealand-children-falling-ill-in-high-numbers-due-to-covid-immunity-debt

McClure, Tess. (2021, July 8). New Zealand children falling ill in high numbers due to Covid 'immunity debt'. *The Guardian*. Retrieved from https://www.theguardian.com/world/2021/jul/08/new-zealand-children-falling-ill-in-high-numbers-due-to-covid-immunity-debt

Donk, Karel. (2020, May 15). Perspectives on the Pandemic – The Bakersfield Doctors. *Karel Donk Channel on Odysee*. Retrieved from Odysee: https://odysee.com/@kareldonk:8/Perspectives-on-the-Pandemic-_-The-Bakersfield-Doctors-_-Episode-6:a

41 — Immunity as a Service – A Subscription-Based Business Model for the Pharmaceutical Industry

Zimbardo, Phillip Dr. (2012, February 20). Ash Conformity Experiment. *Heroic Imagination Project Channel on Youtube*. Retrieved from YouTube: https://www.youtube.com/watch?v=NyDDyT1lDhA

The National Academies of Sciences, Engineering, Medicine. (2016, February 12). *Rapid Medical Countermeasure Response to Infectious Diseases: Enabling Sustainable Capabilities Through Ongoing Public- and Private-Sector Partnerships: Workshop Summary*. Washington (DC): National Academies Press (US). Retrieved from https://www.ncbi.nlm.nih.gov/books/NBK349040/

Engdahl, William. (2010, January 26). European Parliament to Investigate WHO and "Pandemic" Scandal. *Healthcare-in-europe.com*. Retrieved from https://healthcare-in-europe.com/en/news/european-parliament-to-investigate-who-pandemic-scandal.html

Bethge, Philip, Elger, Katrin, et al. (2010, December 3). Reconstruction of a Mass Hysteria: The Swine Flu Panic of 2009. *Spiegel International.* https://www.spiegel.de/international/world/reconstruction-of-a-mass-hysteria-the-swine-flu-panic-of-2009-a-682613.html

Gates, Bill. (2021, March 10). Coronavirus and the money behind vaccines. *Financial Times Channel on YouTube.* Retrieved from YouTube: https://www.youtube.com/watch?v=0BuCt2vtVjc&t=1221s

Lovelace, Berkeley Jr. (2021, April 15). Pfizer CEO says third Covid vaccine dose likely needed within 12 months. *CNBC.* Retrieved from https://www.cnbc.com/2021/04/15/pfizer-ceo-says-third-covid-vaccine-dose-likely-needed-within-12-months.html

Newey, Sarah. (2021, August 7). Variants could be named after star constellations when Greek alphabet runs out, says WHO Covid chief. *The Telegraph.* Retrieved from https://www.telegraph.co.uk/global-health/science-and-disease/variants-could-named-star-constellations-greek-alphabet-runs/

Schrader, Adam. (2021, August 13). Dr. Fauci warns Americans may face having booster shots INDEFINITELY and says fully-vaccinated 'breakthrough' infections could still cause long COVID: FDA approves third dose for those with weakened immune systems. *The Daily Mail.* Retrieved from https://www.dailymail.co.uk/news/article-9889661/Fauci-says-rule-indefinite-COVID-booster-shots-says-one-hopefully-suffice.html

Fauci, Anthony. (2021, August 12). Dr. Fauci: 'Inevitably There Will Be A Time When We Have To Give' Booster Shots. *Today Channel on YouTube.* Retrieved from YouTube: https://www.youtube.com/watch?v=Oz4X4LW5gP0&ab_channel=TODAY

Vucci, Evan. (2021, August 27). Biden Oks booster shots 5 months after 2nd dose. *Boston Globe.* Retrieved from https://www.bostonglobe.com/2021/08/27/world/biden-oks-booster-shots-5-months-after-2nd-dose/

Gomez, Max. (2021, September 10). Moderna Announces Positive Pre-Clinical Data for Single Shot Combining COVID, RSV & Flu Vaccines. *CBS New York.* Retrieved from https://newyork.cbslocal.com/2021/09/10/moderna-single-shot-covid-flu-rsv-vaccine/

Ntc healthcare. (2019). Is Subscription Medicine the Wave of the Future? *Revenue Cycle Solutions.* Retrieved from Ntc Texas: https://web.archive.org/web/20210117183922/https://ntchealthcare.com/resources/is-subscription-medicine-the-wave-of-the-future

Duffy, Kate and Kay, Grace. (2021, May 4). Bill Gates is America's biggest owner of Private farmland, and his 242,000 acres could be split in his divorce. *Business Insider.* Retrieved from https://www.businessinsider.com/bill-gates-land-portfolio-biggest-private-farmland-owner-in-america-2021-1

@APhilosophae. (2021, June 8). Blackrock is buying every single-family house they can find. *Twitter* Retrieved from https://twitter.com/APhilosophae/status/1402434266970140676

Parker, Ceri. (2016, November 12). 8 predictions for the world in 2030. *World Economic Forum.* Retrieved from https://www.weforum.org/agenda/2016/11/8-predictions-for-the-world-in-2030/?utm_content=bufferdda7f&utm_medium=social&utm_source=facebook.com&utm_campaign=buffer

World Economic Forum. (2016, December 9). 8 predictions for the world in 2030. *World Economic Forum on Facebook.* Retrieved from Facebook: https://www.facebook.com/worldeconomicforum/videos/8-predictions-for-the-world-in-2030/10153982130966479/

Wouters, Olivier J. PHD (2020, March 3). Lobbying Expenditures and Campaign Contributions by the Pharmaceutical and Health Product Industry in the United States, 1999-2018. *Jama Internal Medicine*. 180(5):688-697 Retrieved from https://jamanetwork.com/journals/jamainternalmedicine/full article/2762509

Mole, Beth. (2019, January 11). Big Pharma shells out $20B each year to schmooze docs, $6B on drug ads. *ARS Technica* Retrieved from https://arstechnica.com/science/2019/01/healthcare-industry-spends-30b-on-marketing-most-of-it-goes-to-doctors/

Notes

The World Bank. (n.d.). *Hospital beds (per 1,000 people) - Canada*. Retrieved May 28, 2021, from The World Bank: https://data.worldbank.org/indicator/SH.MED.BEDS.ZS?loc ations=CA

Statistics Canada. (2020, July 1). Population estimates on July 1st, by age and sex. *Statistics Canada*. Retrieved from https://www150.statcan.gc.ca/t1/tbl1/en/tv.action?pid=1710 000501&pickMembers%5B0%5D=1.11&pickMembers%5B1 %5D=2.1&cubeTimeFrame.startYear=2016&cubeTimeFrame. endYear=2020&referencePeriods=20160101%2C20200101

Ruechel, J. (2021, January 25). Bystander at the Switch: The Moral Case Against COVID Lockdowns. *www.juliusruechel.com*. Retrieved from https://www.juliusruechel.com/2021/01/bystander-at-switch-moral-case-against.html

@Milhouse_Van_Ho. (2021, April 15). Ontario occupancy rate (tweet – leaked graph). *Twitter*. Retrieved from https://twitter.com/Milhouse_Van_Ho/status/138272453784 2868229

References

Coviddashboard - Data from NHS England). (n.d.). *The UK's response to Covid-19, in facts and figures.* Retrieved May 28, 2021, from The UK's response to Covid-19, in facts and figures: http://www.coviddashboard.live/#beds

Statistics Canada. (n.d.). *Historical Age Pyramid.* Retrieved May 28, 2021, from Statistics Canada: https://www12.statcan.gc.ca/census-recensement/2016/dp-pd/pyramid/pyramid.cfm?type=1&geo1=01

British Medical Journal. (1996, December 7). The Nuremberg Code (1947). *British Medical Journal, 313(7070),* 1448. Retrieved from https://media.tghn.org/medialibrary/2011/04/BMJ_No_7070_Volume_313_The_Nuremberg_Code.pdf

Wikipedia. (n.d.). *Nuremberg Code.* Retrieved May 28, 2021, from Wikipedia: https://en.wikipedia.org/wiki/Nuremberg_Code

About the Author

Julius Ruechel is an independent writer focused on providing perspective on topics essential to the healthy functioning of science and democracy. You can see more of his work on his website at **www.juliusruechel.com**.

Manufactured by Amazon.ca
Bolton, ON

24505133R00153